Intermittent Fasting for Women Over 50:

Detoxify, Regenerate, and Boost Metabolism to Lose Weight and Combat Aging + Anti-Inflammatory Diet Cookbook for Beginners

Lisa Howell

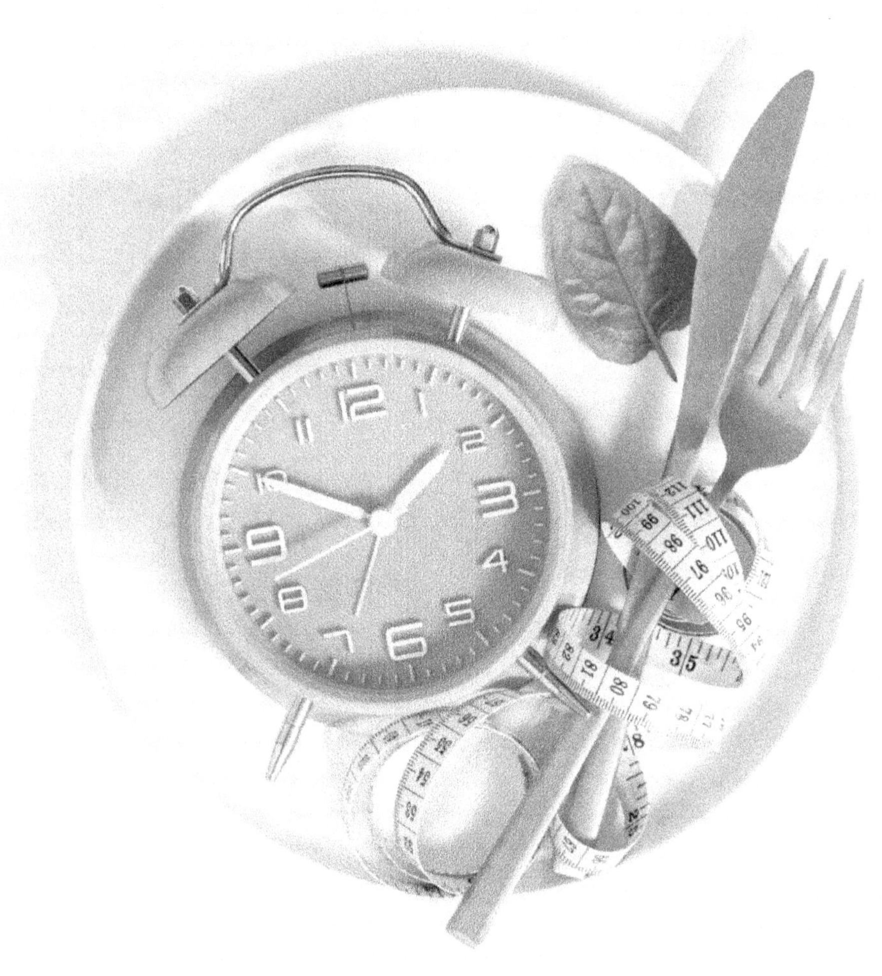

3

Contents

8

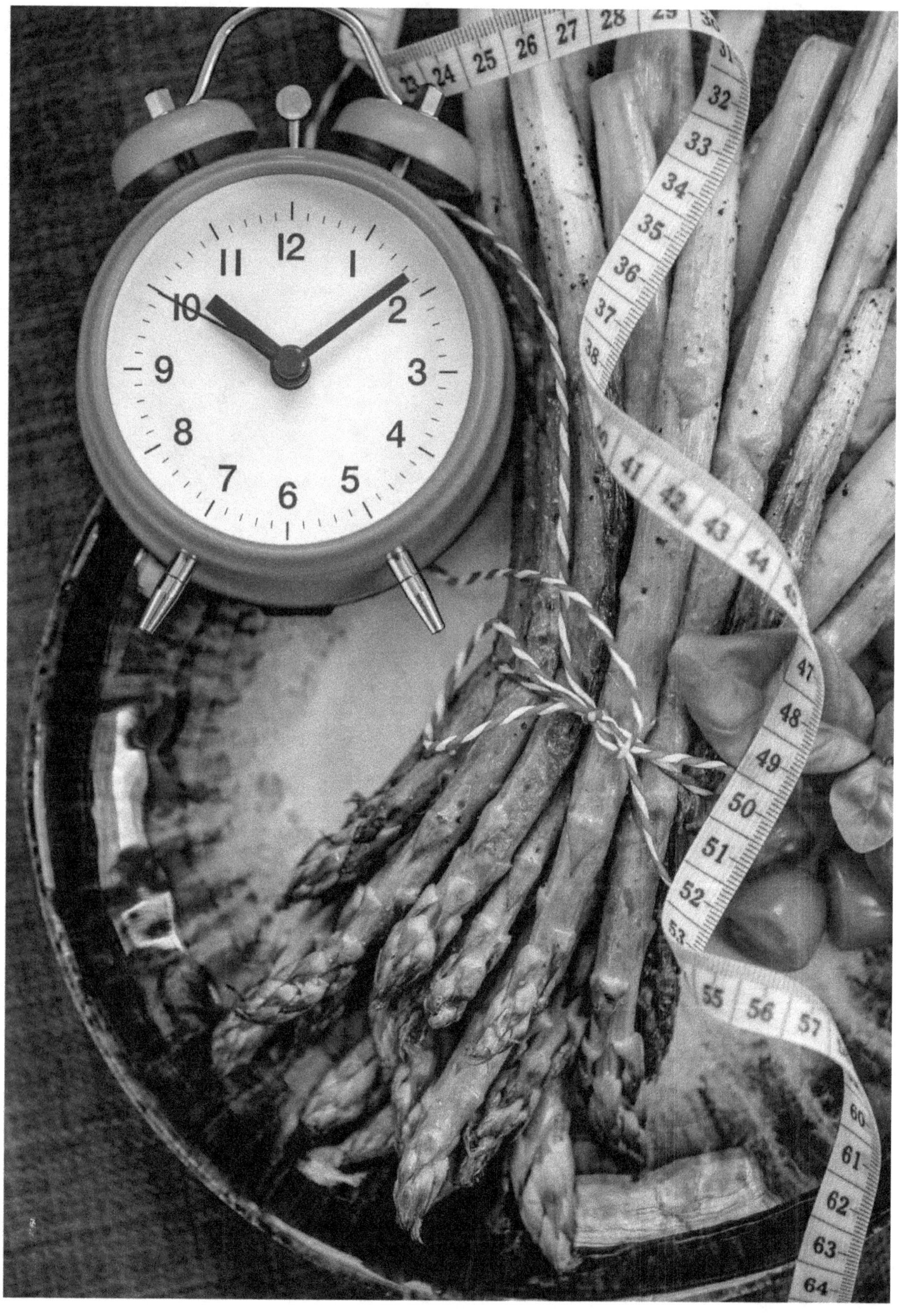

Introduction

Understanding Intermittent Fasting

Intermittent fasting (IF) is not a diet in the conventional sense but rather an eating pattern that cycles between periods of fasting and eating. Unlike traditional diets that focus on what to eat, intermittent fasting focuses on when to eat. This approach has gained significant popularity in recent years due to its simplicity and the compelling body of research supporting its health benefits.

The Basics of Intermittent Fasting

At its core, intermittent fasting involves splitting the day or week into eating and fasting periods. During the fasting periods, you consume very little or no food, while the eating periods allow you to consume meals normally. There are several popular methods of intermittent fasting, each with its own structure and benefits:

The 16/8 Method: This method involves fasting for 16 hours each day and restricting you eating window to 8 hours. For example, you might eat between noon and 8 PM and then fast from 8 PM until noon the next day.

The 5:2 Diet: With this approach, you eat normally for five days of the week and significantly reduce your calorie intake (around 500-600 calories) on the other two days.

Eat-Stop-Eat: This involves fasting for a full 24 hours once or twice a week. For instance, you might fast from dinner one day until dinner the next day.

Alternate Day Fasting: This method involves alternating between days of normal eating and days of fasting or very low-calorie intake.

The Warrior Diet: This approach consists of eating small amounts of raw fruits and vegetables during the day and having one large meal in the evening, typically within a 4-hour eating window.

How Intermittent Fasting Works

Intermittent fasting works by tapping into the body's natural ability to switch between fed and fasted states. When you eat, your body spends several hours processing and absorbing food, during which it uses glucose for energy. In the fasted state, when food intake is minimal or non-existent, the body begins to use stored fat for energy. This metabolic switch can lead to various health benefits, including weight loss, improved metabolic health, and increased cellular repair.

Health Benefits of Intermittent Fasting

Research has shown that intermittent fasting can provide a wide range of health benefits:
Weight Loss and Fat Loss: By reducing the eating window, intermittent fasting can help decrease calorie intake and promote weight loss. It also enhances fat burning by lowering insulin levels.
Improved Metabolic Health: Intermittent fasting can improve insulin sensitivity, lower blood sugar levels, and reduce the risk of type 2 diabetes.
Enhanced Brain Function: Fasting has been shown to support brain health by promoting the production of brain-derived neurotrophic factor (BDNF) and reducing oxidative stress and inflammation.
Increased Longevity: Studies in animals suggest that intermittent fasting can extend lifespan by improving metabolic health and enhancing cellular repair processes.
Better Heart Health: Intermittent fasting can reduce risk factors for heart disease, including blood pressure, cholesterol levels, and triglycerides.

Why Intermittent Fasting is Particularly Beneficial for Women Over 50

For women over 50, intermittent fasting offers several unique advantages:
Hormonal Balance: As women age, hormonal fluctuations can lead to weight gain and metabolic changes. Intermittent fasting can help stabilize hormones like insulin and leptin, aiding in weight management.
Bone Health: Fasting promotes the production of human growth hormone (HGH), which is essential for maintaining bone density and muscle mass.
Enhanced Digestion: Intermittent fasting gives the digestive system a break, which can improve gut health and reduce symptoms of bloating and discomfort.
Mental Clarity and Focus: Many women report increased mental clarity and concentration during fasting periods, which can enhance overall cognitive function.

Practical Considerations and Getting Started

Starting intermittent fasting requires some planning and adjustment. It's important to choose a fasting method that fits your lifestyle and to ease into it gradually. Hydration is crucial during fasting periods, so drink plenty of water, and consider herbal teas or black coffee to help manage hunger. Listening to your body and making adjustments as needed will help ensure that intermittent fasting becomes a sustainable and beneficial part of your routine.

Importance for Women Over 50

Embracing the Golden Years with Vitality

Turning 50 and beyond is a remarkable milestone, bringing with it a wealth of experience, wisdom, and a deeper understanding of life. However, it also comes with unique health challenges and changes in the body that require attention and care. For women over 50, intermittent fasting can be a powerful ally in navigating these changes and enhancing overall well-being.

Hormonal Balance and Metabolic Health

As women age, hormonal shifts become more pronounced, particularly during and after menopause. These changes can lead to a slower metabolism, weight gain, and increased difficulty in maintaining a healthy weight. Intermittent fasting can help regulate insulin levels and improve insulin sensitivity, which are crucial for maintaining a stable metabolism and preventing weight gain. By giving the body regular breaks from food intake, intermittent fasting can also help balance hormones such as leptin and ghrelin, which control hunger and satiety.

Weight Management and Fat Loss

One of the most compelling reasons for women over 50 to consider intermittent fasting is its effectiveness in promoting weight loss and fat loss. With age, the body's metabolic rate naturally slows down, making it easier to gain weight even when maintaining the same eating habits. Intermittent fasting can create a caloric deficit, helping to shed excess pounds and reduce abdominal fat, which is particularly important for reducing the risk of chronic diseases.

Improved Heart Health

Heart disease is a leading health concern for women over 50. Intermittent fasting has been shown to improve various markers of heart health, including lowering blood pressure, reducing LDL cholesterol levels, and decreasing triglycerides. By promoting weight loss and improving metabolic health, intermittent fasting can significantly reduce the risk of heart disease, contributing to a longer and healthier life.

Enhanced Brain Function and Mental Clarity

Aging is often accompanied by concerns about cognitive decline and memory loss. Intermittent fasting supports brain health by stimulating the production of brain-derived neurotrophic factor (BDNF), a protein that promotes the survival of nerve cells and enhances cognitive function. Many women report increased mental clarity and improved focus during fasting periods, which can help maintain sharpness and mental agility.

Supporting Bone and Muscle Health

Maintaining bone density and muscle mass becomes increasingly important with age to prevent conditions like osteoporosis and sarcopenia. Intermittent fasting can support the production of human growth hormone (HGH), which plays a key role in maintaining muscle mass and bone density. Coupled with regular strength training exercises, intermittent fasting can help preserve muscle strength and skeletal health, reducing the risk of fractures and falls.

Improved Digestion and Gut Health

Digestive issues such as bloating, indigestion, and constipation are common concerns for women over 50. Intermittent fasting gives the digestive system regular breaks, which can improve gut health and overall digestion. By allowing the gut time to rest and repair, intermittent fasting can reduce inflammation and promote a healthier balance of gut bacteria, leading to better digestive function and reduced gastrointestinal discomfort.

Increased Energy and Vitality

Many women find that their energy levels fluctuate more with age, often feeling fatigued or sluggish. Intermittent fasting can help stabilize energy levels by preventing the blood sugar spikes and crashes associated with frequent eating. Fasting periods encourage the body to burn fat for fuel, providing a steady source of energy throughout the day. This can lead to increased vitality and a greater sense of well-being.

Emotional and Psychological Benefits

The emotional and psychological benefits of intermittent fasting should not be overlooked. Many women experience a sense of empowerment and control over their eating habits, leading to improved self-esteem and body image. Additionally, the mindfulness required to successfully navigate fasting periods can enhance mental resilience and emotional stability, helping to manage stress and improve overall mental health.

Practical Tips for Starting Intermittent Fasting

For women over 50, starting intermittent fasting should be approached with care and consideration. Here are some practical tips to help you get started:

Choose a Suitable Method: Select a fasting method that fits your lifestyle and daily routine. The 16/8 method is often a good starting point for beginners.

Start Gradually: Ease into intermittent fasting by gradually increasing your fasting window. This allows your body to adjust and helps prevent feelings of deprivation.

Stay Hydrated: Drink plenty of water during fasting periods to stay hydrated and help manage hunger. Herbal teas and black coffee are also good options.

Listen to Your Body: Pay attention to how your body responds to fasting. If you feel weak, dizzy, or excessively hungry, it may be necessary to adjust your fasting schedule.

Focus on Nutrient-Dense Foods: During eating periods, prioritize nutrient-dense foods that provide essential vitamins and minerals. This supports overall health and ensures you get the nutrients your body needs.

Consult Your Healthcare Provider: Before starting intermittent fasting, especially if you have existing health conditions or take medications, consult your healthcare provider to ensure it is safe and appropriate for you.

The History and Origins of Intermittent Fasting

Ancient Practices

Intermittent fasting is far from a modern invention; it is a practice deeply rooted in human history. For thousands of years, our ancestors lived in a world where food scarcity was a common challenge. Hunter-gatherer societies did not have the luxury of regular meals and often went through periods of feast and famine. This natural cycle of eating and fasting was not a choice but a necessity for survival.

During these times, the human body adapted to function efficiently without constant food intake. Fasting periods allowed for the body's metabolic processes to reset, using stored fat for energy when food was not available. This evolutionary adaptation has contributed to the modern understanding of the benefits of intermittent fasting.

Cultural and Religious Fasting Traditions

Throughout history, fasting has also been an integral part of various cultural and religious traditions. These practices are often rooted in spiritual and health beliefs and have been observed by numerous civilizations around the world.

Ancient Greece: The ancient Greeks practiced fasting for both health and spiritual reasons. Philosophers like Pythagoras and Hippocrates advocated fasting as a means to maintain health and enhance mental clarity. Hippocrates, often referred to as the father of medicine, believed that fasting could help the body heal itself by cleansing it of impurities.

Hinduism: In Hinduism, fasting is a common practice observed during various religious festivals and rituals. It is believed to purify the mind and body, promote spiritual growth, and bring one closer to the divine. For example, during the festival of Navratri, many Hindus fast for nine days to honor the goddess Durga.

Buddhism: Buddhist monks and nuns traditionally follow a form of intermittent fasting by refraining from eating after noon. This practice, known as "eating only one meal a day," is intended to aid in meditation, discipline the mind, and reduce attachment to material desires.

Islam: One of the most well-known fasting practices is observed during the holy month of Ramadan in Islam. Muslims fast from dawn to sunset, abstaining from food and drink. This fast, known as sawm, is one of the Five Pillars of Islam and is believed to teach self-discipline, self-control, and empathy for the less fortunate.

Christianity: Fasting has been a significant part of Christian practices, especially during periods such as Lent and Advent. Early Christians fasted to emulate the 40 days Jesus spent fasting in the wilderness. These periods of fasting are seen as times for spiritual reflection, penance, and preparation for significant religious events.

Judaism: In Judaism, fasting is observed on several occasions, most notably on Yom Kippur, the Day of Atonement. Jews fast for 25 hours, seeking repentance and spiritual cleansing. Other fasts, like Tisha B'Av, commemorate historical events and encourage reflection and mourning.

Modern Evolution and Popularity

The practice of intermittent fasting has evolved significantly in modern times, driven by scientific research and the search for effective health and wellness strategies. The resurgence of interest in intermittent fasting can be traced back to the late 20th and early 21st centuries when researchers began to study its physiological effects more rigorously.

Scientific Research: In recent decades, numerous studies have highlighted the benefits of intermittent fasting for weight loss, metabolic health, and longevity. Research by scientists such as Dr. Mark Mattson, a prominent neuroscientist, has shown that intermittent fasting can improve brain function and protect against neurodegenerative diseases.

Popularization: The modern wellness movement has embraced intermittent fasting, popularizing various fasting methods through books, documentaries, and online platforms. Health influencers and medical professionals have contributed to its widespread acceptance by sharing personal success stories and scientific evidence.

Celebrities and Influencers: High-profile endorsements from celebrities and fitness influencers have also played a significant role in the popularity of intermittent fasting. Personalities such as Hugh Jackman, Jennifer Aniston, and Terry Crews have publicly shared their positive experiences with intermittent fasting, inspiring millions to try it themselves.

Health and Wellness Industry: The health and wellness industry has capitalized on the trend by offering a variety of resources, including fasting apps, supplements, and meal planning services. These tools make it easier for individuals to incorporate intermittent fasting into their daily lives and track their progress.

Conclusion

From its ancient roots in survival and religious practices to its modern resurgence driven by scientific research and popular culture, intermittent fasting has a rich and diverse history. This time-tested practice has demonstrated significant benefits for physical, mental, and spiritual health. As we continue to explore and understand the science behind intermittent fasting, it becomes clear that this ancient practice holds valuable insights for achieving optimal health and well-being in the modern world.

The Science Behind Intermittent Fasting

How Intermittent Fasting Works

Intermittent fasting (IF) is more than just a simple eating pattern; it's a powerful tool that leverages the body's natural metabolic processes to promote health and longevity. At its core, intermittent fasting alternates between periods of eating and fasting, allowing the body to cycle between the fed and fasted states. During the fed state, when the body is processing food, insulin levels are higher, and the body stores energy in the form of glycogen and fat. In the fasted state, insulin levels drop, and the body begins to utilize stored energy, primarily from fat reserves.

Metabolic Processes

Glycogen Depletion and Fat Burning

When you eat, your body breaks down carbohydrates into glucose, which enters your bloodstream and provides immediate energy. Any excess glucose is stored in the liver and muscles as glycogen. However, glycogen stores are limited and can be depleted within 24 hours of fasting. Once glycogen stores are exhausted, the body shifts to burning fat for energy, a process known as lipolysis. This transition to fat burning is a key reason why intermittent fasting can be effective for weight loss.

Ketosis

As fasting continues and glycogen stores are depleted, the body may enter a state called ketosis. In ketosis, the liver produces ketones from fatty acids, which can be used as an alternative energy source by the brain and other organs. Ketosis is a metabolic state often associated with the ketogenic diet, but it also occurs naturally during prolonged fasting. Ketones are a more efficient energy source for the brain than glucose and can enhance mental clarity and focus.

Autophagy

Autophagy is a crucial cellular process that is triggered by fasting. It is the body's way of cleaning out damaged cells and regenerating new ones. During autophagy, cells break down and recycle old or dysfunctional components, which helps to remove toxins and repair cellular damage. This process is essential for maintaining cellular health and preventing the accumulation of damaged proteins that can lead to diseases such as cancer and Alzheimer's.

Impact on Hormones and Aging

Insulin and Blood Sugar Regulation

Insulin is a hormone that allows cells to absorb glucose from the bloodstream for energy or storage. Frequent eating, especially of high-carbohydrate foods, keeps insulin levels elevated, which can lead to insulin resistance over time. Insulin resistance is a precursor to type 2 diabetes and is associated with weight gain and metabolic syndrome. Intermittent fasting helps to reduce insulin levels and improve insulin sensitivity, making it easier for the body to regulate blood sugar levels and reduce the risk of diabetes.

Human Growth Hormone (HGH)

Human Growth Hormone (HGH) plays a significant role in growth, metabolism, and muscle strength. Levels of HGH increase during fasting, promoting fat loss and muscle gain. Higher HGH levels also support tissue repair and regeneration, contributing to overall vitality and physical performance. For women over 50, increased HGH can help maintain muscle mass and bone density, which are critical for preventing age-related muscle loss and osteoporosis.

Brain-derived neurotrophic Factor (BDNF)

Intermittent fasting has been shown to increase levels of Brain-Derived Neurotrophic Factor (BDNF), a protein that supports the survival of existing neurons and encourages the growth of new ones. BDNF plays a crucial role in brain plasticity, which is essential for learning and memory. Higher levels of BDNF are associated with improved cognitive function and a reduced risk of neurodegenerative diseases such as Alzheimer's and Parkinson's.

Inflammation and Oxidative Stress

Chronic inflammation and oxidative stress are underlying factors in many age-related diseases, including heart disease, cancer, and dementia. Intermittent fasting helps to reduce inflammation by decreasing the production of pro-inflammatory cytokines and increasing the body's resistance to oxidative stress. This reduction in inflammation and oxidative damage can slow the aging process and improve overall health.

Cellular Repair and Longevity

The activation of autophagy during fasting not only helps with cellular repair but also promotes longevity. By clearing out damaged cells and proteins, the body can function more efficiently and reduce the risk of age-related diseases. Additionally, intermittent fasting has been linked to increased levels of sirtuins, proteins that regulate cellular health, and have been shown to extend lifespan in various organisms. These combined effects contribute to a healthier, longer life.

Conclusion

Intermittent fasting is a scientifically backed approach to health that leverages the body's natural metabolic processes to improve physical and mental well-being. By understanding the mechanisms behind intermittent fasting—such as glycogen depletion, ketosis, and autophagy—and their impact on hormones and aging, we can appreciate how this ancient practice offers profound benefits. For women over 50, intermittent fasting can be a transformative tool, helping to regulate metabolism, support brain health, reduce inflammation, and promote longevity. As you continue reading, you'll discover how to apply this powerful practice to your life effectively and safely.

Effectiveness and Usefulness

Research and Studies

Intermittent fasting (IF) has garnered significant attention in the scientific community, leading to numerous studies that explore its effectiveness and potential health benefits. Research has demonstrated that intermittent fasting can have profound effects on weight management, metabolic health, brain function, and longevity.

Weight Management

One of the most well-documented benefits of intermittent fasting is its ability to promote weight loss and reduce body fat. Studies have shown that intermittent fasting can help individuals lose weight by reducing overall calorie intake and increasing metabolic rate. A review published in the journal *Obesity Reviews* found that intermittent fasting is effective for weight loss, with participants losing an average of 3-8% of their body weight over a 3-24week period.

Metabolic Health

Intermittent fasting has been shown to improve various markers of metabolic health. Research indicates that intermittent fasting can enhance insulin sensitivity, lower blood sugar levels, and reduce inflammation. A study published in *Cell Metabolism* demonstrated that participants who followed an intermittent fasting regimen had improved insulin sensitivity and reduced levels of insulin, blood pressure, and oxidative stress markers.

Brain Function

The benefits of intermittent fasting extend to brain health as well. Animal studies have shown that intermittent fasting can increase the production of brain-derived neurotrophic factor (BDNF), which supports neuron growth and cognitive function. Human studies are still in their early stages, but preliminary results are promising. For example, a study published in *Translational Research* found that intermittent fasting improved cognitive function and reduced markers of inflammation in older adults.

Longevity

Animal studies suggest that intermittent fasting can extend lifespan and delay the onset of age-related diseases. Research on rodents has shown that intermittent fasting can increase lifespan by up to 30-40%. While human studies on longevity are still ongoing, the evidence from animal models provides a compelling case for the potential anti-aging benefits of intermittent fasting.

Short-term vs. Long-term Effects

The effects of intermittent fasting can be observed both in the short term and over the long term, with each timeframe offering distinct benefits and considerations.

Short-term Effects

In the short term, intermittent fasting can lead to rapid weight loss and improvements in metabolic health. Many individuals experience increased energy levels, better focus, and a sense of accomplishment from adhering to a structured eating pattern. Initial weight loss is often due to the reduction in calorie intake and the depletion of glycogen stores, which also leads to a loss of water weight.

Short-term fasting also triggers autophagy, the process of cellular cleanup and repair, which can have immediate benefits for cellular health and function. Additionally, short-term intermittent fasting can help reset eating habits and reduce unhealthy food cravings, leading to more mindful eating practices.

Long-term Effects

Long-term adherence to intermittent fasting can provide sustained weight management and continued improvements in metabolic health. Over time, the body becomes more efficient at burning fat for energy, leading to more stable blood sugar levels and reduced risk of type 2 diabetes. Long-term intermittent fasting can also support cardiovascular health by lowering cholesterol levels, blood pressure, and markers of inflammation.

In terms of longevity and overall health, long-term intermittent fasting may help reduce the risk of chronic diseases such as heart disease, cancer, and neurodegenerative disorders. The ongoing activation of autophagy and reduced oxidative stress contribute to healthier aging and potentially extended lifespan.

Comparisons with Other Diets

Intermittent fasting differs from traditional diets in its approach to eating and fasting periods rather than focusing solely on food choices and calorie restrictions. Here, we compare intermittent fasting with some popular diet plans to highlight its unique benefits and effectiveness.

Calorie-Restricted Diets

Traditional calorie-restricted diets involve reducing daily calorie intake to promote weight loss. While effective, these diets can be challenging to maintain long-term due to constant hunger and the psychological strain of continuous restriction. In contrast, intermittent fasting can be easier to sustain because it focuses on when to eat rather than what to eat, allowing for more flexibility and fewer feelings of deprivation during eating periods.

Low-carb and Ketogenic Diets

Low-carb and ketogenic diets restrict carbohydrate intake to promote fat-burning and ketosis. While both intermittent fasting and ketogenic diets can induce ketosis, intermittent fasting does so without requiring specific macronutrient restrictions. This makes intermittent fasting a more flexible option for those who prefer not to eliminate certain food groups. Combining intermittent fasting with a low-carb or ketogenic diet can enhance the benefits of both approaches.

Plant-Based Diets

Plant-based diets emphasize whole, plant foods and often reduce or eliminate animal products. These diets are associated with numerous health benefits, including improved heart health and reduced risk of chronic diseases. Intermittent fasting can complement a plant-based diet by adding the benefits of improved metabolic health and autophagy.

Together, these approaches can provide a powerful strategy for overall health and well-being.

Conclusion

Intermittent fasting is a highly effective and flexible approach to improving health and managing weight. Scientific research supports its benefits for metabolic health, brain function, and longevity, making it a valuable tool for women over 50. Whether considered in the short term or long term, intermittent fasting offers unique advantages over traditional diets by focusing on when to eat rather than what to eat. As you explore intermittent fasting, you'll find that it can be adapted to suit your lifestyle and dietary preferences, providing a sustainable path to health and vitality.

Why Women Over 50 Should Consider Intermittent Fasting

Health Benefits

As women age, they encounter a range of health challenges that can impact their overall well-being. Intermittent fasting (IF) offers a holistic approach to health, addressing many of these challenges and promoting a healthier, more vibrant life. The health benefits of intermittent fasting are particularly relevant for women over 50, who often face hormonal changes, slower metabolism, and increased risk of chronic diseases.

Hormonal Balance

Menopause brings significant hormonal shifts, including reductions in estrogen and progesterone levels. These changes can lead to weight gain, insulin resistance, and increased risk of metabolic syndrome. Intermittent fasting helps balance insulin levels and improve insulin sensitivity, which can mitigate some of the metabolic changes associated with menopause. Additionally, intermittent fasting promotes the production of human growth hormone (HGH), which supports muscle maintenance and fat metabolism.

Reduced Inflammation

Chronic inflammation is a common issue as we age and is linked to various diseases, including arthritis, heart disease, and diabetes. Intermittent fasting has been shown to reduce markers of inflammation and oxidative stress. By giving the body regular periods of rest from food intake, intermittent fasting helps to lower the levels of inflammatory cytokines and promote a more balanced immune response.

Cardiovascular Health

Heart disease is a leading cause of death among women over 50. Intermittent fasting can improve several risk factors associated with heart disease. Research has shown that intermittent fasting can lower blood pressure, reduce LDL cholesterol levels, and decrease triglycerides. By promoting weight loss and improving metabolic health, intermittent fasting can significantly reduce the risk of cardiovascular diseases.

Weight Management

Maintaining a healthy weight becomes increasingly challenging with age due to hormonal changes and a slower metabolism. Intermittent fasting can be an effective strategy for weight management, offering a sustainable approach to calorie control and fat loss.

Caloric Reduction and Fat Loss

Intermittent fasting naturally reduces calorie intake by limiting the eating window. This caloric deficit, combined with the metabolic boost from fasting, promotes weight loss and fat reduction. Women over 50 often struggle with abdominal fat, which is particularly concerning due to its association with increased health risks. Intermittent fasting targets visceral fat, helping to reduce waist circumference and improve overall body composition.

Improved Metabolism

As we age, our basal metabolic rate (BMR) tends to decline, making it easier to gain weight and harder to lose it. Intermittent fasting can help counteract this decline by boosting metabolism through increased HGH production and improved insulin sensitivity. This metabolic enhancement helps the body burn calories more efficiently, aiding in weight management.

Improved Energy Levels

Many women over 50 experience fluctuations in energy levels, often feeling fatigued or sluggish. Intermittent fasting can help stabilize energy levels and promote a more consistent sense of vitality throughout the day.

Stabilized Blood Sugar Levels

Frequent eating and snacking can lead to blood sugar spikes and crashes, which contribute to feelings of fatigue and lethargy. Intermittent fasting helps to stabilize blood sugar levels by reducing the frequency of insulin release and promoting better glucose control. This leads to more stable energy levels and reduces the likelihood of energy slumps.

Increased Fat Burning

By transitioning the body into a fat-burning state, intermittent fasting provides a steady source of energy from fat reserves. This sustained energy supply can help maintain higher energy levels throughout the day, improving overall stamina and reducing feelings of tiredness.

Enhanced Mental Clarity

Cognitive decline is a concern for many women as they age. Intermittent fasting offers benefits that extend to brain health, enhancing mental clarity and cognitive function.

Boosted Brain Function

Intermittent fasting increases the production of brain-derived neurotrophic factor (BDNF), a protein that supports neuron growth and cognitive function. Higher levels of BDNF are associated with improved memory, learning, and mental clarity. This can be particularly beneficial for women over 50 who may experience age-related cognitive changes.

Neuroprotective Effects

Research suggests that intermittent fasting can protect the brain from neurodegenerative diseases such as Alzheimer's and Parkinson's. The process of autophagy, triggered by fasting, helps clear out damaged cells and proteins, reducing the risk of cognitive decline. Additionally, the reduction in inflammation and oxidative stress further supports brain health.

Enhanced Focus and Concentration

Many individuals report improved focus and concentration during fasting periods. This mental clarity is likely due to the stable energy supply from fat burning and the reduction in blood sugar fluctuations. For women over 50, this enhanced cognitive function can improve productivity and overall quality of life.

Conclusion

Intermittent fasting offers a range of compelling benefits for women over 50, from promoting hormonal balance and reducing inflammation to aiding in weight management and enhancing mental clarity. As the body undergoes various changes with age, intermittent fasting provides a flexible and sustainable approach to maintaining health and vitality. By embracing this powerful practice, women over 50 can navigate the challenges of aging with greater ease and confidence, leading to a healthier and more fulfilling life.

Potential Risks and Precautions

Common Concerns

Intermittent fasting (IF) has gained popularity for its numerous health benefits, but it's essential to approach it with awareness of potential risks and precautions, especially for women over 50. Understanding common concerns can help mitigate risks and ensure a safe and effective fasting experience.

Nutrient Deficiencies

One of the primary concerns with intermittent fasting is the potential for nutrient deficiencies. Restricting eating windows can sometimes lead to inadequate intake of essential vitamins and minerals. Women over 50 need to be particularly mindful of calcium, vitamin D, and magnesium to support bone health, as well as iron and B vitamins for overall vitality.

Electrolyte Imbalance

Extended fasting periods can lead to imbalances in electrolytes such as sodium, potassium, and magnesium, which are crucial for maintaining muscle function and fluid balance. Symptoms of electrolyte imbalance include fatigue, muscle cramps, and dizziness. It's important to ensure adequate hydration and consider electrolyte supplementation if necessary.

Eating Disorders

For individuals with a history of eating disorders or disordered eating patterns, intermittent fasting might trigger unhealthy behaviors. The restrictive nature of fasting can lead to binge eating during eating windows or exacerbate obsessive thoughts about food and body image. It's vital to approach intermittent fasting with a healthy mindset and be aware of these potential psychological risks.

Digestive Issues

Some people may experience digestive issues such as constipation, bloating, or gastrointestinal discomfort when starting intermittent fasting. These issues often arise from changes in eating patterns or reduced fiber intake during fasting periods. Gradually transitioning into intermittent fasting and ensuring a balanced diet can help mitigate these digestive concerns.

Medical Conditions and Considerations

Certain medical conditions require special consideration when practicing intermittent fasting. It's crucial to understand how fasting may interact with existing health issues to avoid complications.

Diabetes and Blood Sugar Control

For individuals with diabetes, especially type 1 diabetes or those on insulin, intermittent fasting can pose significant risks. Fasting affects blood sugar levels and insulin sensitivity, which can lead to hypoglycemia (low blood sugar) or hyperglycemia (high blood sugar) if not carefully managed. Diabetics need to consult with their healthcare provider before starting intermittent fasting.

Thyroid Conditions

Women with thyroid conditions, such as hypothyroidism or hyperthyroidism, should exercise caution with intermittent fasting. Fasting can influence hormone levels and metabolic rate, potentially impacting thyroid function. Regular monitoring and adjustments to medication may be necessary under the guidance of a healthcare professional.

Gastrointestinal Disorders

Individuals with gastrointestinal disorders such as irritable bowel syndrome (IBS), acid reflux, or inflammatory bowel disease (IBD) need to be cautious with intermittent fasting. Fasting can exacerbate symptoms or disrupt digestive health. A tailored approach, possibly with shorter fasting periods or modifications to the fasting protocol, may be needed.

Heart Conditions

For those with heart conditions, such as hypertension or arrhythmias, intermittent fasting can have both beneficial and adverse effects. While fasting may improve cardiovascular markers, abrupt changes in diet and electrolyte balance can pose risks. Close monitoring and consultation with a cardiologist are recommended.

Consulting with Healthcare Providers

Before starting intermittent fasting, it is crucial for women over 50 to consult with healthcare providers. Professional guidance ensures that intermittent fasting is safe and tailored to individual health needs.

Individual Health Assessment

A comprehensive health assessment by a healthcare provider can help identify potential risks and determine the most suitable fasting regimen. This assessment should include a review of medical history, current medications, and any pre-existing conditions.

Personalized Fasting Plan

Based on the health assessment, a healthcare provider can help develop a personalized fasting plan that aligns with individual health goals and needs. This plan may involve choosing the appropriate fasting method (e.g., 16/8, 5:2), adjusting fasting periods, and incorporating nutrient-dense foods to prevent deficiencies.

Monitoring and Adjustments

Regular monitoring is essential to track the effects of intermittent fasting on health markers such as blood sugar levels, blood pressure, and weight. Healthcare providers can make necessary adjustments to the fasting regimen or medications to ensure optimal health outcomes.

Regular Check-ins

Regular check-ins with healthcare providers are essential to monitor progress and address any concerns that may arise during intermittent fasting. These check-ins allow for ongoing support, guidance, and adjustments to the fasting regimen as needed. Open communication with healthcare providers ensures that any changes in health status or medication management are appropriately addressed.

Comprehensive Health Management

Intermittent fasting should be viewed as one component of a comprehensive approach to health management. Alongside fasting, it's essential to prioritize other aspects of health, including regular physical activity, adequate sleep, stress management, and a balanced diet rich in nutrient-dense foods. Incorporating these lifestyle factors can further enhance the benefits of intermittent fasting and promote overall well-being.

Conclusion

While intermittent fasting offers numerous health benefits, it's essential to approach it with awareness of potential risks and precautions, especially for women over 50. By understanding common concerns, considering specific medical conditions, and consulting with healthcare providers, women can ensure a safe and effective fasting experience. Regular monitoring, personalized guidance, and comprehensive health management contribute to maximizing the benefits of intermittent fasting while minimizing any potential risks. With proper precautions in place, intermittent fasting can be a valuable tool for improving health and well-being in women over 50, empowering them to lead healthier and more fulfilling lives.

Types of Intermittent Fasting

Intermittent fasting (IF) encompasses a variety of fasting regimens, each with its own unique approach to alternating between eating and fasting periods. Understanding the different types of intermittent fasting can help women over 50 choose the method that best fits their lifestyle, preferences, and health goals.

16/8 Method

The 16/8 method, often referred to as the Leangains protocol, has gained significant popularity in the realm of intermittent fasting due to its simplicity and flexibility. This approach involves splitting the day into two distinct periods: a fasting window and an eating window.

During the fasting period, which typically lasts for 16 hours, individuals abstain from consuming any calories, relying solely on water, herbal tea, or black coffee to help manage hunger and maintain hydration. The fasting window begins after the last meal of the day and extends until the first meal of the following day.

The eating window, on the other hand, spans 8 hours during which individuals consume all their daily calories and nutrients. This window often starts around midday and ends in the early evening, though the timing can be adjusted to suit individual preferences and lifestyle constraints.

One of the key benefits of the 16/8 method is its adaptability to various schedules and lifestyles. Whether you're an early riser who prefers breakfast or a night owl who enjoys late dinners, the eating window can be tailored to accommodate your unique needs. Additionally, the simplicity of the approach makes it easy to implement and sustain over the long term.

Beyond its convenience, the 16/8 method has been associated with several potential health benefits. Research suggests that intermittent fasting, including the 16/8 approach, may help regulate blood sugar levels, improve insulin sensitivity, promote fat loss, and even support cellular repair and autophagy.

However, it's important to note that the effectiveness of the 16/8 method can vary depending on individual factors such as age, gender, activity level, and overall health status. Additionally, while intermittent fasting can be a safe and effective strategy for many people, it may not be suitable for everyone, particularly those with certain medical conditions or dietary needs.

As with any dietary or lifestyle change, it's advisable to consult with a healthcare professional before starting intermittent fasting, especially if you have any underlying health concerns or are taking medications. Additionally, listening to your body and adjusting the approach as needed is key to finding a sustainable fasting routine that works for you.

5:2 Diet

The 5:2 diet, also known as the Fast Diet, has gained popularity as another approach to intermittent fasting. This method involves alternating between regular eating days and fasting days throughout the week. On fasting days, individuals limit their calorie intake to approximately 500-600 calories, while on non-fasting days, they can eat normally without any specific restrictions.

One of the key features of the 5:2 diet is its flexibility, allowing individuals to choose which days they want to fast based on their schedule and preferences. Some people prefer to spread out their fasting days evenly throughout the week, while others may prefer to fast on consecutive days. This flexibility can make the 5:2 diet more manageable and sustainable for some individuals compared to other forms of intermittent fasting.

During fasting days, individuals often opt for small, nutrient-dense meals to help manage hunger and maintain energy levels. These meals may include lean proteins, vegetables, fruits, and healthy fats to provide essential nutrients while keeping calorie intake low. Some common choices for fasting day meals include salads, soups, vegetable stir-fries, and protein-rich snacks like Greek yogurt or cottage cheese.

On non-fasting days, individuals are encouraged to eat a balanced diet that includes a variety of nutrient-rich foods to support overall health and well-being. This may include lean proteins, whole grains, fruits, vegetables, and healthy fats. By allowing for unrestricted eating on non-fasting days, the 5:2 diet can help prevent feelings of deprivation and promote a healthy relationship with food.

Research on the 5:2 diet suggests that it may offer several potential health benefits, including weight loss, improved metabolic health, and reduced risk factors for chronic diseases such as heart disease and diabetes. Additionally, intermittent fasting has been shown to promote cellular repair processes and increase levels of brain-derived neurotrophic factor (BDNF), a protein that supports brain health and cognitive function.

However, it's important to note that the 5:2 diet may not be suitable for everyone, particularly those with certain medical conditions or dietary needs. Pregnant or breastfeeding women, individuals with a history of eating disorders, and those with diabetes or other metabolic conditions should consult with a healthcare professional before starting any fasting regimen.

As with any dietary approach, the 5:2 diet should be personalized to fit individual needs and goals. It's important to listen to your body, stay hydrated, and make informed choices about food quality and portion sizes. Working with a registered dietitian or nutritionist can also provide guidance and support in implementing the 5:2 diet safely and effectively.

Eat-Stop-Eat

Eat-Stop-Eat is a form of intermittent fasting that has gained popularity, particularly due to the work of author Brad Pilon. This approach involves fasting for a full 24 hours once or twice a week, with no calorie consumption during the fasting period. For example, an individual might choose to fast from dinner one day until dinner the following day, effectively going without food for a full day.

One of the key aspects of Eat-Stop-Eat is its simplicity. Unlike some other forms of intermittent fasting that involve daily fasting windows or alternating fasting days, Eat-Stop-Eat requires only one or two days of fasting per week. This can make it an attractive option for individuals who prefer a more straightforward approach to fasting.

During the fasting period, individuals consume only non-caloric beverages such as water, herbal tea, or black coffee to help manage hunger and stay hydrated. While fasting for a full 24 hours may require greater discipline and willpower, many people find that the structure and predictability of Eat-Stop-Eat make it easier to adhere to over the long term.

On non-fasting days, individuals are free to eat normally without any specific restrictions. This flexibility allows for unrestricted eating, which can help prevent feelings of deprivation and make it easier to stick to the fasting regimen. It also means that individuals can enjoy their favorite foods and meals without guilt, knowing that they have a designated fasting day coming up.

Research on intermittent fasting, including the Eat-Stop-Eat approach, suggests that it may offer several potential health benefits. These include weight loss, improved metabolic health, increased insulin sensitivity, and even longevity. Fasting for extended periods may also promote cellular repair processes and autophagy, which can have positive effects on overall health and well-being.

However, it's important to note that fasting for 24 hours may not be suitable for everyone, particularly those with certain medical conditions or dietary needs. Pregnant or breastfeeding women, individuals with a history of eating disorders, and those with diabetes or other metabolic conditions should consult with a healthcare professional before starting any fasting regimen.

As with any dietary approach, it's essential to listen to your body, stay hydrated, and make informed choices about food quality and quantity. Experimenting with different fasting protocols and finding what works best for you is key to developing a sustainable fasting routine that supports your health and well-being.

Alternate Day Fasting

Alternate day fasting is a form of intermittent fasting characterized by alternating between fasting days and non-fasting days. This approach has gained attention in recent years for its potential benefits for weight loss and metabolic health.

During fasting days, individuals typically consume very few calories, if any at all. Some variations of alternate-day fasting allow for a small meal or snack to help manage hunger, while others involve complete calorie restriction. Fasting days often involve consuming only non-caloric beverages such as water, herbal tea, or black coffee to help suppress appetite and stay hydrated.

On non-fasting days, individuals are free to eat normally without any specific restrictions. This flexibility allows for enjoyment of favorite foods and meals without the need to restrict calories or food choices. However, it's important to maintain a balanced diet on non-fasting days to ensure adequate intake of essential nutrients.

One of the key challenges of alternate day fasting is the frequency of fasting days, which can make it more difficult for some individuals to adhere to compared to other forms of intermittent fasting. The transition between fasting and non-fasting days may also require adjustment, both physically and mentally, as the body adapts to changes in calorie intake and meal timing.

Research on alternate-day fasting suggests that it may offer significant benefits for weight loss, metabolic health, and longevity. Studies have shown that alternate-day fasting can lead to reductions in body weight, body fat, and markers of inflammation, as well as improvements in insulin sensitivity and cardiovascular health.

However, it's important to note that alternate-day fasting may not be suitable for everyone, particularly those with certain medical conditions or dietary needs. Pregnant or breastfeeding women, individuals with a history of eating disorders, and those with diabetes or other metabolic conditions should consult with a healthcare professional before starting any fasting regimen.

As with any dietary approach, it's essential to listen to your body, stay hydrated, and make informed choices about food quality and quantity. Experimenting with different fasting protocols and finding what works best for you is key to developing a sustainable fasting routine that supports your health and well-being.

Choosing the Right Method for You

When selecting an intermittent fasting method, it's essential to consider various factors, including lifestyle, preferences, health status, and goals.

Lifestyle and Schedule

Choose a fasting method that aligns with your daily routine and commitments. For example, the 16/8 method may be more suitable for those with regular work hours, while alternate-day fasting may be challenging for individuals with unpredictable schedules.

Dietary Preferences

Consider your dietary preferences and eating habits when selecting a fasting method. If you prefer larger meals or specific meal timing, choose a method that allows for flexibility and accommodates your preferences.

Health Considerations

Take into account any underlying health conditions or medical concerns when choosing an intermittent fasting method. Consult with healthcare providers to ensure that the selected method is safe and appropriate for your individual health needs.

Long-Term Sustainability

Select a fasting method that you can maintain over the long term. Sustainability is key to success with intermittent fasting, so choose a method that feels manageable and enjoyable for you.

Experimentation and Adaptation

Be open to experimenting with different fasting methods and adjusting as needed based on your experiences and results. What works for one person may not work for another, so be willing to adapt and find the approach that best suits you.

Crafting Your Eating Plan

Crafting a personalized eating plan is essential for women over 50 embarking on an intermittent fasting journey. This chapter will explore the nutritional needs of women in this age group, provide sample meal plans tailored to intermittent fasting, discuss strategies for balancing macronutrients and micronutrients, and emphasize the importance of hydration and electrolyte balance.

Nutritional Needs for Women Over 50

As women age, their nutritional needs evolve to support overall health and well-being. Key considerations include maintaining bone health, supporting hormone balance, managing weight, and reducing the risk of chronic diseases such as heart disease and osteoporosis.

Calcium and Vitamin D

Calcium and vitamin D are critical for bone health, especially for women over 50 who are at higher risk of osteoporosis. Good dietary sources of calcium include dairy products, leafy greens, tofu, and fortified foods. Vitamin D can be obtained from sunlight exposure and foods such as fatty fish, egg yolks, and fortified dairy products.

Protein

Protein is essential for maintaining muscle mass, supporting metabolism, and promoting satiety during fasting periods. Women over 50 should aim to include protein-rich foods in their eating plan, such as lean meats, poultry, fish, eggs, dairy products, legumes, and tofu.

Healthy Fats

Healthy fats provide essential fatty acids and support hormone production and brain health. Incorporate sources of healthy fats such as avocados, nuts, seeds, olive oil, and fatty fish like salmon into your meals.

Fiber
Fiber is crucial for digestive health, regulating blood sugar levels, and promoting satiety. Include fiber-rich foods such as fruits, vegetables, whole grains, legumes, nuts, and seeds in your eating plan to support overall health and well-being.

Sample Meal Plans

Intermittent fasting meal plans can vary based on individual preferences and fasting schedules. Here are two sample meal plans tailored to different fasting methods:

16/8 Method Meal Plan
Eating Window: 12:00 PM - 8:00 PM
12:00 PM (Breakfast/Lunch):
Spinach and feta omelette
Whole grain toast
Mixed berries
3:00 PM (Snack):
Greek yogurt with honey and almonds
6:30 PM (Dinner):
Grilled chicken breast
Quinoa salad with mixed vegetables
Steamed broccoli
5:2 Diet Meal Plan
Fasting Days: 500-600 calorie meals
Breakfast:
Veggie omelette with spinach, tomatoes, and mushrooms (200 calories)
Lunch:
Grilled chicken salad with mixed greens, cucumber, and vinaigrette dressing (300 calories)
Dinner:
Baked salmon with roasted vegetables (400 calories)
Balancing Macronutrients and Micronutrients
Balancing macronutrients (carbohydrates, protein, and fat) and micronutrients (vitamins and minerals) is essential for meeting nutritional needs and supporting overall health.

This table provides a brief overview of some common intermittent fasting methods, each with its own unique approach to fasting and eating patterns.

#	Fasting Method	Description
1	16/8 Method	Fast for 16 hours and eat during an 8-hour window each day. Commonly involves skipping breakfast and having meals between 12 PM and 8 PM.
2	5:2 Diet	Eat normally for 5 days of the week and restrict calorie intake to 500-600 calories on two non-consecutive days.
3	Eat-Stop-Eat	Fast for a full 24 hours once or twice a week, usually by skipping dinner one day and fasting until dinner the next day.
4	Alternate Day Fasting	Alternate between regular eating days and fasting days, where you consume little to no calories every other day.
5	OMAD (One Meal a Day)	Consume all calories within a single meal, fasting for the remaining 23 hours of the day.
6	Warrior Diet	Fast for 20 hours and eat within a 4-hour window, typically consuming one large meal in the evening.

Macronutrients:

Carbohydrates: Choose complex carbohydrates such as whole grains, fruits, and vegetables for sustained energy and fiber.

Protein: Include lean protein sources to support muscle maintenance and satiety.

Fat: Incorporate healthy fats from sources like nuts, seeds, avocados, and olive oil for hormone balance and brain health.

Micronutrients:

Vitamins: Aim for a variety of colorful fruits and vegetables to obtain essential vitamins such as vitamin C, vitamin A, and vitamin K.

Minerals: Include mineral-rich foods like leafy greens, nuts, seeds, and dairy products to support bone health, muscle function, and overall vitality.

Hydration and Electrolytes

Proper hydration and electrolyte balance are crucial during intermittent fasting to support overall health and well-being.

Water: Drink plenty of water throughout the day to stay hydrated, especially during fasting periods.

Electrolytes: Ensure adequate intake of electrolytes such as sodium, potassium, and magnesium. Incorporate electrolyte-rich foods like leafy greens, bananas, nuts, and seeds into your meals, or consider using electrolyte supplements if needed.

Conclusion

Intermittent fasting offers a range of options to fit different lifestyles, preferences, and health goals. Whether you prefer the simplicity of the 16/8 method, the flexibility of the 5:2 diet, the discipline of Eat-Stop-Eat, or the structure of alternate-day fasting, there is a fasting method to suit your needs. By considering factors such as lifestyle, dietary preferences, health considerations, and long-term sustainability, women over 50 can choose the intermittent fasting method that aligns with their individual needs and preferences, empowering them to achieve their health and wellness goals.

Emphasizing the Role of Physical Activity

Physical activity plays a crucial role in supporting overall health and well-being, especially when combined with intermittent fasting. Engaging in regular exercise can enhance the benefits of fasting, promote weight management, support muscle maintenance, and improve cardiovascular health. Incorporating a variety of exercises into your routine can help you achieve a well-rounded fitness regimen that complements your fasting schedule.

Strength Training: Building Muscle and Boosting Metabolism
Strength training is an essential component of any exercise program, particularly for women over 50. As we age, we naturally lose muscle mass, which can lead to a slower metabolism and decreased strength. Strength training exercises, such as weightlifting, resistance band exercises, and bodyweight exercises, help build and maintain muscle mass, increase bone density, and improve overall strength and function. By incorporating strength training into your routine, you can boost your metabolism, enhance fat loss, and support healthy aging.

Cardio Workouts: Improving Heart Health and Stamina
Cardiovascular exercise is vital for maintaining heart health, improving endurance, and burning calories. Including cardio workouts in your exercise routine can help support weight loss, enhance cardiovascular function, and increase overall energy levels. Examples of cardio exercises include brisk walking, jogging, cycling, swimming, and aerobics. Aim to incorporate at least 150 minutes of moderate-intensity cardio exercise or 75 minutes of vigorous-intensity cardio exercise each week, spread out over several sessions, to reap the full benefits of cardiovascular activity.

Flexibility and Balance Exercises: Enhancing Mobility and Stability
Flexibility and balance exercises are essential for maintaining mobility, preventing injuries, and promoting functional independence as we age. These exercises focus on improving joint flexibility, range of motion, and proprioception (body awareness), helping to reduce the risk of falls and injuries. Examples of flexibility and balance exercises include yoga, tai chi, Pilates, and stretching routines. Incorporating these exercises into your routine can improve posture, reduce stiffness, and enhance overall mobility and stability.

Sample Exercise Routines

Strength Training Routine:

Warm-up: 5-10 minutes of light cardio (e.g., brisk walking, jumping jacks)

Strength Exercises: Perform 2-3 sets of 8-12 repetitions of each exercise.

Squats

Lunges

Chest presses

Rows

Shoulder presses

Bicep curls

Tricep dips

Cool-down: 5-10 minutes of stretching exercises targeting major muscle groups.

Cardio Workout Routine:

Warm-up: 5-10 minutes of light cardio (e.g., jogging in place, high knees)

Cardio Exercises: Choose one or more cardio activities and perform for 20-30 minutes.

Brisk walking or jogging

Cycling

Swimming

Dancing

Jump rope

Cool-down: 5-10 minutes of gentle stretching to reduce muscle tension and promote flexibility.

Flexibility and Balance Routine:

Warm-up: 5-10 minutes of dynamic stretching (e.g., arm circles, leg swings)

Flexibility Exercises: Hold each stretch for 20-30 seconds, focusing on major muscle groups and areas of tightness.

Hamstring stretch

Quadriceps stretch

Chest stretch

Shoulder stretch

Calf stretch

Balance Exercises: Perform balance exercises such as single-leg stands, heel-to-toe walks, and balance board exercises for 5-10 minutes.

Cool-down: 5-10 minutes of relaxation exercises (e.g., deep breathing, gentle yoga poses).

Mindset and Resilience

Harnessing the Psychological Benefits of Fasting
Intermittent fasting offers more than just physical benefits; it can also have profound effects on mental well-being. Adopting a positive mindset and cultivating resilience are essential components of a successful fasting journey for women over 50.
Building Mental Toughness
Fasting requires discipline and mental strength to overcome challenges and stick to your fasting schedule. Building mental toughness involves developing resilience, perseverance, and self-control. By reframing challenges as opportunities for growth and focusing on long-term goals, women can cultivate mental toughness and navigate obstacles with confidence and determination.
Mindfulness and Meditation: Cultivating Inner Peace
Mindfulness and meditation practices can complement intermittent fasting by promoting relaxation, reducing stress, and enhancing self-awareness. Incorporating mindfulness techniques, such as deep breathing exercises, body scans, and mindful eating, can help women over 50 stay present and attentive during fasting periods. Meditation practices, such as guided visualization, loving-kindness meditation, and gratitude meditation, can promote emotional well-being and resilience, fostering a positive mindset and inner peace.

Conclusion

Incorporating a variety of exercises into your routine can complement your intermittent fasting regimen and support overall health and well-being. Strength training helps build and maintain muscle mass, boosting metabolism and promoting healthy aging. Cardio workouts improve heart health, endurance, and calorie burn. Flexibility and balance exercises enhance mobility, stability, and functional independence. By combining these different types of exercises and following sample exercise routines, women over 50 can create a well-rounded fitness program that enhances the benefits of intermittent fasting and promotes a healthy and active lifestyle.

How to Regenerate and Rejuvenate

Unveiling the Power of Cellular Autophagy

At the core of intermittent fasting's ability to regenerate and rejuvenate lies the intricate process of cellular autophagy. This biological mechanism serves as a cellular clean-up crew, breaking down and recycling damaged or dysfunctional components within cells. Intermittent fasting acts as a catalyst for autophagy, prompting cells to initiate this vital process. As a result, toxins are expelled, damage is repaired, and cells undergo renewal, ultimately leading to improved cellular function and overall health.

Delving Deeper into Anti-Aging Benefits

Intermittent fasting emerges as a potent tool for combating the aging process, offering a myriad of benefits that extend beyond mere physical appearance. By promoting cellular regeneration, reducing inflammation, and bolstering metabolic health, intermittent fasting stands as a formidable ally against the relentless march of time. Fasting-induced autophagy plays a pivotal role in this anti-aging arsenal, as it works tirelessly to repair DNA damage, enhance mitochondrial function, and fortify cellular resilience. Moreover, intermittent fasting amplifies the production of growth hormone, a vital catalyst for tissue repair and regeneration. Through these mechanisms, intermittent fasting exerts profound anti-aging effects, empowering individuals to defy the passage of time and maintain vitality as they age.

Nurturing Longevity with Intermittent Fasting

Emerging research unveils intermittent fasting as a promising strategy for extending lifespan and promoting longevity. By activating longevity pathways within cells, fasting sets the stage for enhanced cellular health and resilience. Key among these pathways are sirtuins, a family of proteins that wield significant influence over cellular processes associated with aging and longevity. Intermittent fasting acts as a potent activator of sirtuins, bolstering their activity and thereby safeguarding against age-related decline. Through this intricate interplay of cellular mechanisms, intermittent fasting emerges as a beacon of hope for those seeking to prolong their lifespan and embrace a future filled with vitality and vigor.

Embracing the Fountain of Youth

In the quest for regeneration and rejuvenation, intermittent fasting stands as a beacon of hope, offering a pathway to enhanced cellular health, anti-aging benefits, and longevity. Through the lens of cellular autophagy, we witness the remarkable capacity of fasting to ignite cellular renewal and fortify resilience. The anti-aging prowess of intermittent fasting becomes evident as we delve into its ability to repair DNA, enhance mitochondrial function, and stimulate growth hormone production. Moreover, the promise of longevity beckons, as intermittent fasting activates longevity pathways within cells, paving the way for a future filled with vitality and vigor. As we unlock the secrets of cellular regeneration and rejuvenation, intermittent fasting emerges as a timeless ally in the pursuit of a life well-lived, offering the promise of a brighter, healthier tomorrow.

Understanding Natural Detox Processes

Detoxification is a natural and ongoing process that occurs in the body to eliminate toxins and waste products. Key organs involved in detoxification include the liver, kidneys, lungs, skin, and digestive system. These organs work together to neutralize and eliminate harmful substances, ensuring the body remains balanced and healthy. Intermittent fasting can support the body's natural detox processes by providing periods of rest and allowing energy to be redirected towards detoxification pathways.

Supporting Liver Function

The liver plays a central role in detoxification, filtering toxins from the blood and metabolizing them into less harmful substances for elimination. Intermittent fasting can support liver function by reducing the burden of continuous digestion and allowing the liver to focus on detoxification. Additionally, fasting promotes the production of enzymes involved in detoxification pathways, enhancing the liver's ability to neutralize toxins effectively. To further support liver health during fasting, it's essential to stay hydrated, consume nutrient-dense foods, and limit exposure to environmental toxins.

Detox-Friendly Foods and Supplements

Incorporating detox-friendly foods and supplements into your diet can enhance the body's natural detoxification processes. Key nutrients and compounds that support detoxification include antioxidants, vitamins, minerals, fiber, and phytonutrients. Foods such as leafy greens, cruciferous vegetables, berries, citrus fruits, garlic, turmeric, and ginger are rich in detoxifying nutrients and can be included in your diet during fasting periods. Additionally, certain supplements, such as milk thistle, dandelion root, N-acetylcysteine (NAC), and glutathione, can support liver health and enhance detoxification.

Detoxification and cleansing are vital processes that support overall health and well-being. Intermittent fasting can enhance the body's natural detox processes by providing periods of rest and promoting liver function. By incorporating detox-friendly foods and supplements into your diet, you can further support detoxification and optimize the benefits of fasting. As you embark on your intermittent fasting journey, prioritize liver health, and nourish your body with nutrient-dense foods that support detoxification. By supporting your body's natural detox processes, you can promote optimal health and vitality, ensuring that you look and feel your best at any age.

Monitoring Progress and Adjusting Plans:
Tracking Results: The Importance of Monitoring

Tracking progress is essential for gauging the effectiveness of your intermittent fasting regimen and ensuring that you're moving closer to your health and wellness goals. There are various methods for monitoring progress, including keeping a food journal, tracking fasting windows, recording measurements such as weight and body measurements, and noting changes in energy levels, mood, and overall well-being. By regularly monitoring your progress, you can identify trends, track improvements, and make informed decisions about adjusting your fasting plan as needed.

Adapting to Changes in Your Body

As you continue with intermittent fasting, it's essential to listen to your body and be attuned to any changes or signals it may be sending. Pay attention to how you feel during fasting periods and adjust your eating plan accordingly. If you experience increased hunger, fatigue, or other symptoms, consider modifying your fasting schedule, adjusting meal timing, or incorporating more nutrient-dense foods into your diet. Additionally, be mindful of any changes in your body composition, energy levels, and overall health, and adapt your fasting plan to accommodate these changes.

Dealing with Setbacks: Overcoming Challenges

Setbacks are a natural part of any journey, including intermittent fasting. It's essential to approach setbacks with resilience, patience, and a positive mindset. If you veer off track or encounter obstacles along the way, don't be discouraged. Instead, view setbacks as learning opportunities and opportunities for growth. Identify the factors that led to the setback, whether it's stress, social situations, or cravings, and develop strategies for overcoming these challenges in the future. Remember that intermittent fasting is a flexible and adaptable approach to health and wellness, and setbacks should not deter you from pursuing your goals.

Conclusion

Monitoring progress and adjusting your intermittent fasting plan are essential components of a successful and sustainable fasting journey. By tracking results, adapting to changes in your body, and dealing with setbacks with resilience and positivity, you can navigate the ups and downs of intermittent fasting with confidence and determination. Remember that intermittent fasting is a journey, and it's normal to experience setbacks and challenges along the way. By staying focused on your goals, listening to your body, and being flexible in your approach, you can overcome obstacles, make progress, and achieve long-term success with intermittent fasting.

Success Stories and Examples

Real-life Experiences: Stories of Transformation

Real-life success stories provide inspiration and motivation for women over 50 who are embarking on their intermittent fasting journey. Hearing about the experiences of others who have achieved positive results through fasting can help individuals feel encouraged and empowered to pursue their own health and wellness goals. These stories highlight the diverse ways in which intermittent fasting can impact lives, from weight loss and improved energy levels to enhanced mental clarity and overall well-being.

Case Studies: Illustrating the Power of Intermittent Fasting

Case studies offer a closer look at the tangible benefits of intermittent fasting through the lens of individual experiences. By examining specific examples of individuals who have successfully implemented fasting into their lives, readers can gain insights into the practical application of fasting principles and strategies. Case studies provide valuable information about the challenges faced, the methods employed, and the outcomes achieved, offering a roadmap for others to follow on their own fasting journey.

Inspiration and Motivation: Fueling the Fire Within

Inspiration and motivation are essential ingredients for sustaining long-term success with intermittent fasting. Hearing about the achievements of others, witnessing their transformations, and recognizing the possibilities for personal growth and change can ignite a sense of purpose and determination within individuals. Whether it's through before-and-after photos, testimonials, or personal anecdotes, sharing stories of success can fuel the fire within and propel women over 50 towards their own goals with renewed enthusiasm and commitment.

Maintaining a Healthy Lifestyle Beyond Fasting

Sustainable Healthy Habits: Building a Foundation for Wellness

While intermittent fasting can be a powerful tool for improving health and well-being, it's essential to maintain sustainable healthy habits beyond fasting periods. Sustainable habits form the foundation of a healthy lifestyle and contribute to long-term success and well-being. These habits include eating a balanced diet rich in whole foods, staying hydrated, getting regular exercise, prioritizing sleep, managing stress, and nurturing social connections. By incorporating these habits into your daily routine, you can support your overall health and well-being both during and beyond fasting periods.

Integrating Fasting with Everyday Life: Finding Balance and Flexibility

Integrating intermittent fasting into your everyday life requires finding a balance that works for you and your lifestyle. While fasting can offer numerous health benefits, it's essential to approach it with flexibility and adaptability. Consider your daily schedule, commitments, and personal preferences when determining your fasting protocol. Experiment with different fasting methods, meal timings, and eating patterns to find what feels sustainable and manageable for you. By integrating fasting into your everyday life in a way that aligns with your needs and preferences, you can maintain consistency and continuity in your fasting practice over the long term.

Continuous Learning and Growth: Embracing the Journey

Embarking on a journey of health and wellness is an ongoing process of learning and growth. As you navigate the ups and downs of intermittent fasting and healthy living, embrace the opportunity for continuous learning and self-improvement. Stay curious, explore new ideas and approaches, and be open to adapting your habits and routines as needed. Educate yourself about nutrition, exercise, and lifestyle factors that contribute to overall well-being, and seek out resources, support, and guidance to help you on your journey. By approaching your health journey with a growth mindset and a commitment to lifelong learning, you can cultivate resilience, adaptability, and empowerment to thrive in all areas of your life.

In conclusion, intermittent fasting for women over 50 offers a multifaceted approach to health and well-being, encompassing physical, mental, and emotional benefits. Through the exploration of various topics such as the history and origins of intermittent fasting, the science behind it, its effectiveness and usefulness, and the specific considerations for women over 50, we've uncovered a wealth of information and insights.

Intermittent fasting has ancient roots and has evolved into a popular wellness practice with demonstrated benefits for weight management, metabolic health, cognitive function, and longevity. For women over 50, intermittent fasting can be particularly beneficial, offering opportunities to support hormonal balance, manage weight, boost energy levels, and enhance overall vitality.

However, it's crucial to approach intermittent fasting with a holistic perspective, considering not only the fasting protocol but also factors such as nutrition, exercise, mindset, resilience, detoxification, and continuous learning and growth. By incorporating nutrient-dense foods, engaging in regular physical activity, cultivating a positive mindset, supporting detoxification processes, and embracing opportunities for personal development, women over 50 can maximize the benefits of intermittent fasting and maintain a healthy lifestyle beyond fasting periods.

Ultimately, intermittent fasting is not just about restricting food intake but about nourishing the body, mind, and soul in a way that promotes optimal health and well-being. It's a journey of self-discovery, empowerment, and transformation, offering the opportunity to thrive at every stage of life. As women over 50 embrace the principles of intermittent fasting and integrate them into their lives with intention and mindfulness, they can unlock the full potential of this powerful wellness practice and experience the joy of living a vibrant, fulfilling life.

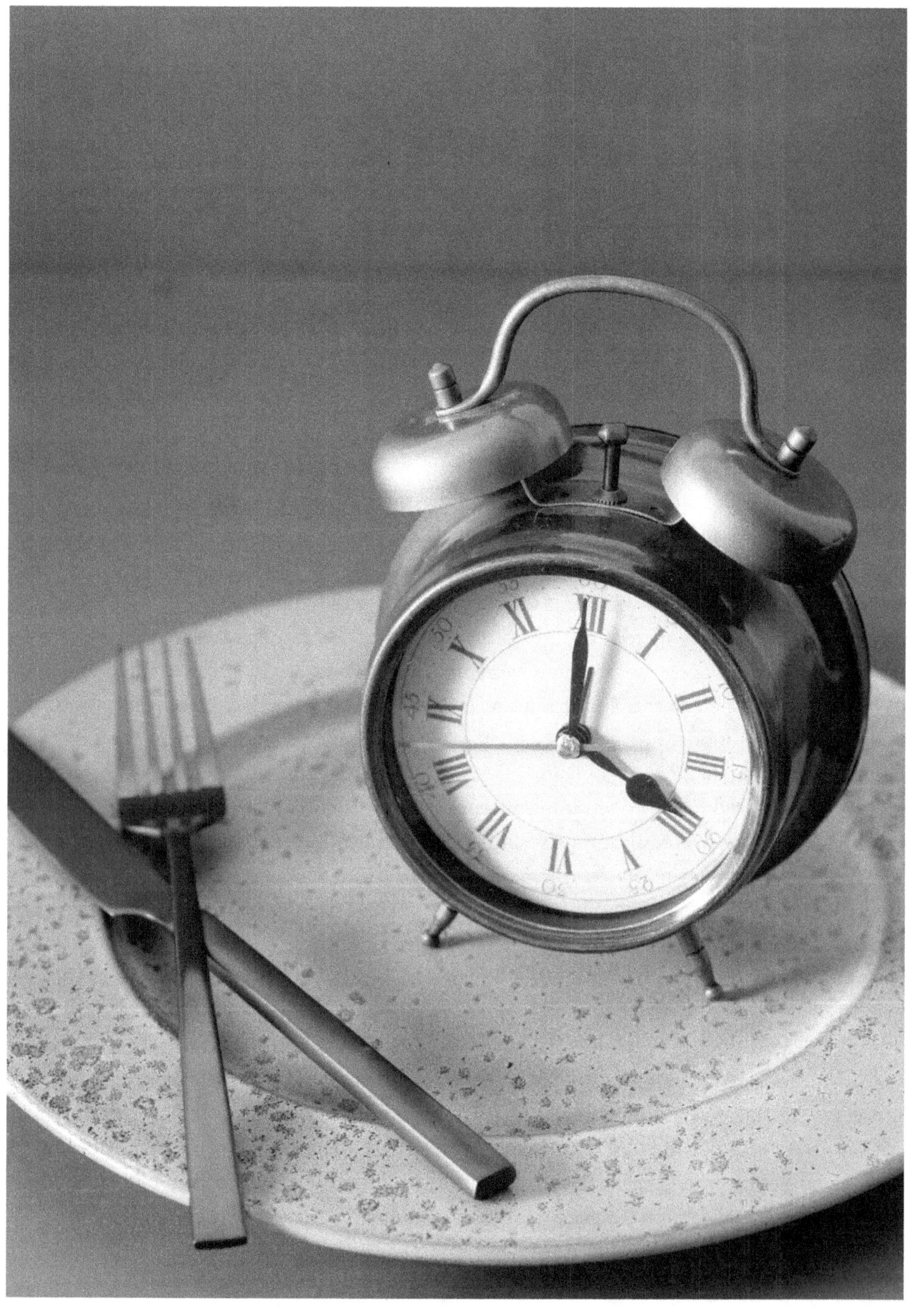

Recipes

1. Greek Yogurt and Berry Parfait

Ingredients:

1 cup plain Greek yogurt (8oz)

1/2 cup mixed berries (strawberries, blueberries, raspberries)

1 tablespoon chia seeds

1 tablespoon sliced almonds

1/4 teaspoon vanilla extract (optional)

Preparation:

In a bowl, mix Greek yogurt with vanilla extract (if using).

Layer the yogurt in a glass or bowl.

Add a layer of mixed berries on top of the yogurt.

Sprinkle chia seeds and sliced almonds over the berries.

Nutrition Facts:

Nutrient	Amount
Calories	250
Protein	20g
Total Fat	10g
Sugars	10g
Carbs	20g
Calcium	200mg
Potassium	300mg

Practical Tips:

Use fresh or frozen berries. Preparation Time: 5 minutes

2. Spinach and Feta Stuffed Chicken Breast

Ingredients:

1 boneless, skinless chicken breast (7oz)

1/2 cup fresh spinach, chopped

1/4 cup feta cheese, crumbled

1 tablespoon olive oil

Salt and pepper to taste

Preparation:

Preheat the oven to 375°F.

Butterfly the chicken breast by slicing it horizontally to create a pocket.

In a bowl, mix chopped spinach and feta cheese.

Stuff the chicken breast with the spinach and feta mixture.

Secure with toothpicks if necessary.

Season the chicken with salt and pepper.

Heat olive oil in an oven-safe skillet over medium-high heat.

Sear the chicken for 2-3 minutes on each side until golden brown.

Transfer the skillet to the oven and bake for 15-20 minutes until the chicken is cooked through.

Remove from the oven and let rest for 5 minutes before serving.

Nutrition Facts:

Nutrient	Amount
Calories	300
Protein	35g
Total Fat	15g
Sugars	1g
Carbs	2g
Calcium	150mg
Iron	2mg

3. Quinoa and Vegetable Stir-Fry

Ingredients:

1/2 cup cooked quinoa (3.5oz)

1/2 cup bell peppers, sliced

1/2 cup broccoli florets

1/4 cup carrots, julienned

1 tablespoon low-sodium soy sauce

1 teaspoon sesame oil

1 clove garlic, minced

1/2 teaspoon grated ginger

Preparation:

Cook quinoa according to package instructions.

Heat sesame oil in a large skillet over medium-high heat.

Add garlic and ginger, sauté for 1 minute.

Add bell peppers, broccoli, and carrots. Stir-fry for 5-7 minutes until vegetables are tender-crisp.

Add cooked quinoa and soy sauce, stirring to combine.

Cook for an additional 2 minutes until heated through.

Serve immediately.

Nutrition Facts:

Nutrient	Amount
Calories	280
Protein	9g
Total Fat	8g
Sugars	4g
Carbs	42g
Potassium	500mg
Vitamin C	60mg

Practical Tips:

Add tofu or chicken for additional protein. Preparation Time: 20 minutes

4. Avocado and Shrimp Salad

Ingredients:

1/2 ripe avocado, diced

3.5 oz cooked shrimp

1 cup mixed salad greens

1/4 cup cherry tomatoes, halved

1 tablespoon lemon juice

1 tablespoon olive oil

Salt and pepper to taste

Preparation:

In a large bowl, combine mixed salad greens, diced avocado, cherry tomatoes, and cooked shrimp.

In a small bowl, whisk together lemon juice, olive oil, salt, and pepper.

Drizzle the dressing over the salad and toss to combine.

Serve immediately.

Nutrition Facts:

Nutrient	Amount
Calories	300
Protein	20g
Total Fat	22g
Sugars	2g
Carbs	10g
Potassium	700mg
Vitamin C	30mg

Practical Tips:

Use pre-cooked shrimp for convenience.

Preparation Time: 10 minutes

5. Lentil and Vegetable Soup

Ingredients:

1/2 cup lentils, rinsed (3.5oz)

1/2 cup diced tomatoes

1/4 cup diced carrots

1/4 cup diced celery

1/4 cup diced onion

2 cloves garlic, minced

1 tablespoon olive oil

2 cups vegetable broth

1 teaspoon cumin

Salt and pepper to taste

Preparation:

Heat olive oil in a large pot over medium heat.

Add onions, carrots, celery, and garlic. Sauté for 5 minutes until vegetables are softened.

Add diced tomatoes, lentils, vegetable broth, cumin, salt, and pepper.

Bring to a boil, then reduce heat and simmer for 25-30 minutes until lentils are tender.

Adjust seasoning if necessary and serve hot.

Nutrition Facts:Practical Tips:

Nutrient	Amount
Calories	250
Protein	12g
Total Fat	7g
Sugars	6g
Carbs	36g
Iron	4mg
Potassium	600mg

Use a pressure cooker to reduce cooking time. Preparation Time: 35 minutes

6. Grilled Salmon with Asparagus

Ingredients:

6 oz salmon fillet

1/2 tablespoon olive oil

1/2 lemon, sliced

1 garlic clove, minced

1 cup asparagus, trimmed

Salt and pepper to taste

Preparation:

Preheat the grill to medium-high heat.

Brush salmon fillet with olive oil and season with salt, pepper, and minced garlic.

Place salmon on the grill, skin-side down, and cook for 4-5 minutes per side, or until it flakes easily with a fork.

While salmon is cooking, grill asparagus for 3-4 minutes until tender.

Serve the salmon with a squeeze of lemon juice and grilled asparagus on the side.

Nutrition Facts:

Nutrient	Amount
Calories	350
Protein	34g
Total Fat	20g
Sugars	2g
Carbs	8g
Omega-3	1.8g
Vitamin D	570 IU

Practical Tips:
Use a grill pan if outdoor grilling is not available.
Preparation Time: 15 minutes

7. Turkey and Avocado Lettuce Wraps

Ingredients:

3oz cooked turkey breast, sliced

1/2 avocado, sliced

2 large lettuce leaves

1/4 cup shredded carrots

1 tablespoon hummus

Salt and pepper to taste

Preparation:

Lay out the lettuce leaves on a plate.

Spread hummus evenly on each leaf.

Layer turkey slices, avocado, and shredded carrots on the lettuce.

Season with salt and pepper.

Roll up the lettuce leaves to form wraps and serve.

Nutrition Facts:

Nutrient	Amount
Calories	200
Protein	20g
Total Fat	12g
Sugars	2g
Carbs	10g
Fiber	5g
Vitamin K	50mcg

Practical Tips:
Secure with toothpicks to keep wraps together.
Preparation Time: 10 minutes

8. Egg and Vegetable Breakfast Muffins

Ingredients:

2 large eggs

1/4 cup chopped spinach

1/4 cup diced bell peppers

1/4 cup diced tomatoes

1 tablespoon milk

Salt and pepper to taste

Preparation:

Preheat oven to 350°F.

In a bowl, whisk together eggs, milk, salt, and pepper.

Add chopped spinach, bell peppers, and tomatoes to the egg mixture.

Pour the mixture into a greased muffin tin, filling each cup about 2/3 full.

Bake for 15-20 minutes or until the muffins are set and golden brown.

Let cool slightly before serving.

Nutrition Facts:

Nutrient	Amount
Calories	150
Protein	12g
Total Fat	10g
Sugars	3g
Carbs	5g
Iron	2mg
Vitamin A	3000 IU

Practical Tips:

Store in the fridge for up to 3 days for a quick breakfast.

Preparation Time: 25 minutes

9. Chickpea and Tomato Salad

Ingredients:

1 cup canned chickpeas, rinsed and drained

1/2 cup cherry tomatoes, halved

1/4 cup diced cucumber

1/4 cup red onion, diced

1 tablespoon olive oil

1 tablespoon lemon juice

Salt and pepper to taste

Preparation:

In a large bowl, combine chickpeas, cherry tomatoes, cucumber, and red onion.

Drizzle with olive oil and lemon juice.

Season with salt and pepper.

Toss to combine and serve.

Nutrition Facts:

Nutrient	Amount
Calories	220
Protein	8g
Total Fat	8g
Sugars	4g
Carbs	30g
Fiber	10g
Vitamin C	20mg

Practical Tips:

Add fresh herbs like parsley or cilantro for extra flavor.

Preparation Time: 10 minutes

10. Cauliflower Rice Stir-Fry

Ingredients:

1 cup cauliflower rice

1/2 cup mixed vegetables (peas, carrots, bell peppers)

1 egg, beaten

1 tablespoon soy sauce

1 tablespoon sesame oil

1 clove garlic, minced

1/2 teaspoon grated ginger

Preparation:

Heat sesame oil in a large skillet over medium-high heat.

Add garlic and ginger, sauté for 1 minute.

Add mixed vegetables and cook for 3-4 minutes until tender.

Push vegetables to one side of the skillet and add the beaten egg, scrambling until fully cooked.

Add cauliflower rice and soy sauce, stirring to combine with vegetables and egg.

Cook for another 2-3 minutes until heated through.

Serve immediately.

Nutrition Facts:

Nutrient	Amount
Calories	180
Protein	8g
Total Fat	10g
Sugars	4g
Carbs	14g
Fiber	4g
Vitamin A	3500 IU

Practical Tips: Use frozen cauliflower rice to save time.

11. Grilled Chicken and Quinoa Salad

Ingredients:

1 chicken breast (6oz)

1/2 cup cooked quinoa (3.5oz)

1 cup mixed greens

1/4 cup cherry tomatoes, halved

1/4 cup cucumber, diced

1 tablespoon olive oil

1 tablespoon balsamic vinegar

Salt and pepper to taste

Preparation:

Season the chicken breast with salt and pepper.

Grill the chicken over medium-high heat for 6-7 minutes per side until fully cooked.

Slice the grilled chicken and set aside.

In a large bowl, combine mixed greens, cherry tomatoes, cucumber, and cooked quinoa.

In a small bowl, whisk together olive oil and balsamic vinegar.

Toss the salad with the dressing and top with grilled chicken slices.

Serve immediately.

Nutrition Facts:

Nutrient	Amount
Calories	400
Protein	35g
Total Fat	14g
Sugars	4g
Carbs	30g
Fiber	6g

Practical Tips: Use pre-cooked quinoa to save time. Preparation Time: 20 minutes

12. Baked Cod with Lemon and Dill

Ingredients:

1 cod fillet (6 oz)

1 tablespoon olive oil

1 lemon, sliced

1 tablespoon fresh dill, chopped

Salt and pepper to taste

Preparation:

Preheat the oven to 375°F.

Place the cod fillet on a baking sheet lined with parchment paper.

Drizzle olive oil over the cod and season with salt, pepper, and chopped dill.

Arrange lemon slices on top of the cod.

Bake for 15-20 minutes until the cod is opaque and flakes easily with a fork.

Serve with a side of steamed vegetables.

Nutrition Facts:

Nutrient	Amount
Calories	250
Protein	28g
Total Fat	12g
Sugars	1g
Carbs	6g
Potassium	700mg
Vitamin D	400 IU

Practical Tips:

Use fresh or frozen cod.

Preparation Time: 25 minutes

13. Mediterranean Chickpea Bowl

Ingredients:

1/2 cup canned chickpeas, rinsed and drained (3.5 oz)

1/4 cup diced cucumber

1/4 cup cherry tomatoes, halved

1/4 cup red onion, diced

1/4 cup feta cheese, crumbled

1 tablespoon olive oil

1 tablespoon lemon juice

Salt and pepper to taste

Preparation:

In a large bowl, combine chickpeas, cucumber, cherry tomatoes, red onion, and feta cheese.

Drizzle with olive oil and lemon juice.

Season with salt and pepper.

Toss to combine and serve immediately.

Nutrition Facts:

Add olives for extra Mediterranean flavor.

Preparation Time: 10 minutes

Nutrient	Amount
Calories	300
Protein	12g
Total Fat	16g
Sugars	5g
Carbs	28g
Fiber	8g

14. Veggie Omelette

Ingredients:

2 large eggs

1/4 cup diced bell peppers

1/4 cup diced onions

1/4 cup spinach, chopped

1 tablespoon milk

1 tablespoon olive oil

Salt and pepper to taste

Preparation:

In a bowl, whisk together eggs, milk, salt, and pepper.

Heat olive oil in a non-stick skillet over medium heat.

Add bell peppers and onions, sauté for 3-4 minutes until softened.

Add spinach and cook for another 1-2 minutes until wilted.

Pour the egg mixture into the skillet, spreading it evenly.

Cook for 2-3 minutes until the eggs are set, then fold the omelette in half.

Serve immediately.

Nutrition Facts:

Nutrient	Amount
Calories	200
Protein	14g
Total Fat	15g
Sugars	2g
Carbs	6g
Iron	2mg
Vitamin A	2500 IU

Practical Tips:

Use a non-stick skillet for easy cooking. Preparation Time: 10 minutes

15. Shrimp and Avocado Salad

Ingredients:

3.5oz cooked shrimp

1/2 avocado, diced

1 cup mixed greens

1/4 cup cherry tomatoes, halved

1/4 cup cucumber, diced

1 tablespoon olive oil

1 tablespoon lime juice

Salt and pepper to taste

Preparation:

In a large bowl, combine mixed greens, shrimp, avocado, cherry tomatoes, and cucumber.

In a small bowl, whisk together olive oil, lime juice, salt, and pepper.

Drizzle the dressing over the salad and toss to combine.

Serve immediately.

Nutrition Facts:

Nutrient	Amount
Calories	250
Protein	20g
Total Fat	15g
Sugars	3g
Carbs	10g
Potassium	700mg
Vitamin C	20mg

Practical Tips:

Use pre-cooked shrimp for convenience.

Preparation Time: 10 minutes

16. Zucchini Noodles with Pesto

Ingredients:

2 medium zucchinis

1/4 cup pesto sauce

1 tablespoon olive oil

1/4 cup cherry tomatoes, halved

1 tablespoon grated Parmesan cheese

Salt and pepper to taste

Preparation:

Use a spiralizer to turn the zucchinis into noodles.

Heat olive oil in a large skillet over medium heat.

Add zucchini noodles and cook for 3-4 minutes until slightly tender.

Add pesto sauce and cherry tomatoes, tossing to combine.

Cook for another 2 minutes until heated through.

Season with salt and pepper.

Serve topped with grated Parmesan cheese.

Nutrition Facts:

Nutrient	Amount
Calories	250
Protein	6g
Total Fat	20g
Sugars	5g
Carbs	16g
Fiber	4g
Vitamin C	35mg

Practical Tips:

Use pre-made pesto sauce for convenience.

Preparation Time: 15 minutes

17. Tuna and White Bean Salad

Ingredients:

1 can tuna in water (5 oz), drained

1/2 cup canned white beans, rinsed and drained

1/4 cup red onion, diced

1/4 cup cherry tomatoes, halved

1 tablespoon olive oil

1 tablespoon lemon juice

1 tablespoon fresh parsley, chopped

Salt and pepper to taste

Preparation:

In a large bowl, combine tuna, white beans, red onion, cherry tomatoes, and parsley.

Drizzle with olive oil and lemon juice.

Season with salt and pepper.

Toss to combine and serve immediately.

Nutrition Facts:
Practical Tips:
Use solid white albacore tuna for the best texture.
Preparation Time: 10 minutes

Nutrient	Amount
Calories	280
Protein	25g
Total Fat	12g
Sugars	2g
Carbs	20g
Fiber	6g
Vitamin C	0,5mg

18. Spaghetti Squash with Marinara Sauce

Ingredients:

1 small spaghetti squash (about 2 lbs)

1 cup marinara sauce

1 tablespoon olive oil

1/4 cup grated Parmesan cheese

1/4 cup fresh basil, chopped

Salt and pepper to taste

Preparation:

Preheat the oven to 400°F.

Cut the spaghetti squash in half lengthwise and remove the seeds.

Drizzle with olive oil and season with salt and pepper.

Place squash halves cut-side down on a baking sheet and bake for 40-45 minutes until tender.

Use a fork to scrape out the squash into strands.

Heat marinara sauce in a saucepan over medium heat.

Serve spaghetti squash topped with marinara sauce, Parmesan cheese, and fresh basil.

Nutrition Facts:

Nutrient	Amount
Calories	250
Protein	8g
Total Fat	12g
Sugars	10g
Carbs	30g
Fiber	6g
Vitamin A	1500 IU

Practical Tips:

Use a sharp knife to carefully cut the spaghetti squash. Preparation Time: 50 minutes

19. Turkey and Spinach Stuffed Bell Peppers

Ingredients:

1 large bell pepper

4 oz ground turkey

1 cup fresh spinach, chopped

1/4 cup diced tomatoes

1/4 cup quinoa, cooked

1 tablespoon olive oil

1/4 cup shredded mozzarella cheese

Salt and pepper to taste

Preparation:

Preheat the oven to 375°F.

Cut the top off the bell pepper and remove the seeds.

In a skillet, heat olive oil over medium heat and cook ground turkey until browned.

Add chopped spinach and diced tomatoes, cooking until spinach is wilted.

Stir in cooked quinoa and season with salt and pepper.

Stuff the bell pepper with the turkey mixture.

Place the stuffed pepper in a baking dish and top with shredded mozzarella cheese.

Bake for 25-30 minutes until the pepper is tender and the cheese is melted.

Nutrition Facts:

Nutrient	Amount
Calories	300
Protein	25g
Total Fat	15g
Sugars	6g
Carbs	20g
Fiber	5g
Vitamin C	100mg

Practical Tips:
Use different colored bell peppers for a visually appealing dish.

20. Cauliflower and Chickpea Curry

Ingredients:

1 cup cauliflower florets

1/2 cup canned chickpeas, rinsed and drained

1/2 cup diced tomatoes

1/4 cup coconut milk

1 tablespoon curry powder

1 tablespoon olive oil

1 clove garlic, minced

1/2 teaspoon grated ginger

Salt and pepper to taste

Preparation:

Heat olive oil in a large skillet over medium heat.

Add garlic and ginger, sauté for 1 minute.

Add cauliflower florets and cook for 5-7 minutes until slightly tender.

Add chickpeas, diced tomatoes, coconut milk, and curry powder.

Stir to combine and bring to a simmer.

Cook for an additional 10 minutes until cauliflower is tender and the sauce has thickened.

Preparation Time: 20 minutes

Season with salt and pepper.

Nutrition Facts:

Nutrient	Amount
Calories	280
Protein	8g
Total Fat	14g
Sugars	7g
Carbs	30g
Fiber	10g
Iron	3mg

Practical Tips: Serve with a side of brown rice or quinoa.

21. Lentil and Vegetable Soup

Ingredients:

1/2 cup dried lentils, rinsed
1 carrot, diced
1 celery stalk, diced
1/2 onion, diced
1 clove garlic, minced
1 tablespoon olive oil
4 cups vegetable broth
1/2 teaspoon cumin
1/2 teaspoon paprika
Salt and pepper to taste
1 cup spinach leaves

Preparation:

Heat olive oil in a large pot over medium heat.

Add onion, carrot, and celery, and cook until vegetables are tender, about 5 minutes.

Add garlic and cook for another minute.

Stir in lentils, vegetable broth, cumin, paprika, salt, and pepper.

Bring to a boil, then reduce heat and simmer for 25-30 minutes, until lentils are tender.

Stir in spinach leaves and cook until wilted, about 2 minutes.

Serve hot.

Nutrition Facts:

Nutrient	Amount
Calories	350
Protein	30g
Total Fat	15g
Sugars	4g
Carbs	20g
Fiber	5g
Vitamin C	120mg

22. Chicken and Broccoli Stir-Fry

Ingredients:

6 oz chicken breast, sliced thin

1 cup broccoli florets

1/2 bell pepper, sliced

1/2 onion, sliced

2 tablespoons soy sauce

1 tablespoon sesame oil

1 clove garlic, minced

1/2 teaspoon ginger, grated

1 tablespoon sesame seeds

Salt and pepper to taste

Preparation:

Heat sesame oil in a large skillet over medium-high heat.

Add garlic and ginger, and cook for 1 minute.

Add chicken slices and cook until browned, about 5-6 minutes.

Add broccoli, bell pepper, and onion, and stir-fry for 5-7 minutes until vegetables are tender.

Stir in soy sauce and cook for another 2 minutes.

Sprinkle with sesame seeds before serving.

Nutrition Facts:

Nutrient	Amount
Calories	350
Protein	30g
Total Fat	15g
Sugars	4g
Carbs	20g
Fiber	5g
Vitamin C	120mg

Practical Tips:

Serve with a side of brown rice or quinoa. Preparation Time: 20 minutes

23. Greek Yogurt Parfait

Ingredients:

1 cup Greek yogurt

1/4 cup fresh blueberries

1/4 cup fresh strawberries, sliced

1 tablespoon chia seeds

1 tablespoon honey (optional)

2 tablespoons granola

Preparation:

In a bowl or parfait glass, layer half of the Greek yogurt.

Add half of the blueberries, strawberries, and chia seeds.

Repeat the layers with the remaining yogurt, berries, and chia seeds.

Drizzle with honey if desired and top with granola.

Serve immediately.

Nutrition Facts:
Practical Tips:
Use seasonal fruits for variety.

Nutrient	Amount
Calories	300
Protein	20g
Total Fat	7g
Sugars	20g
Carbs	40g
Fiber	6g
Calcium	200mg

Preparation Time: 5 minutes

24. Avocado and Egg Salad

Ingredients:

1 ripe avocado, diced

2 hard-boiled eggs, chopped

1 tablespoon lemon juice

1 tablespoon olive oil

1 tablespoon fresh parsley, chopped

Salt and pepper to taste

Preparation:

In a bowl, combine diced avocado and chopped eggs.

Drizzle with lemon juice and olive oil.

Add chopped parsley, salt, and pepper.

Gently mix all ingredients together.

Serve on its own or on a bed of mixed greens.

Nutrition Facts:
Practical Tips:
Serve with whole grain toast for a heartier meal.
Preparation Time: 10 minutes

Nutrient	Amount
Calories	350
Protein	12g
Total Fat	30g
Sugars	1g
Carbs	14g
Fiber	10g
Vitamin E	4mg

25. Shrimp and Mango Salad

Ingredients:

4 oz cooked shrimp

1/2 mango, diced

1/2 avocado, diced

2 cups mixed greens

1 tablespoon lime juice

1 tablespoon olive oil

1/4 cup red onion, thinly sliced

Salt and pepper to taste

Preparation:

In a large bowl, combine cooked shrimp, diced mango, diced avocado, mixed greens, and red onion.

In a small bowl, whisk together lime juice, olive oil, salt, and pepper.

Drizzle the dressing over the salad and toss to combine.

Serve immediately.

Nutrition Facts:

Practical Tips:

Use pre-cooked shrimp for a quicker preparation.

Preparation Time: 10 minutes

Nutrient	Amount
Calories	300
Protein	18g
Total Fat	20g
Sugars	10g
Carbs	20g
Fiber	8g
Vitamin C	60mg

26. Turkey and Vegetable Skewers

Ingredients:

6 oz turkey breast, cut into chunks

1 bell pepper, cut into chunks

1 zucchini, sliced

1 red onion, cut into chunks

2 tablespoons olive oil

1 teaspoon dried oregano

1 teaspoon smoked paprika

Salt and pepper to taste

Preparation:

Preheat grill to medium-high heat.

Thread turkey, bell pepper, zucchini, and onion onto skewers.

In a small bowl, mix olive oil, oregano, paprika, salt, and pepper.

Brush skewers with the olive oil mixture.

Grill skewers for 10-12 minutes, turning occasionally, until turkey is cooked through and vegetables are tender.

Serve hot.

Nutrition Facts:

Nutrient	Amount
Calories	280
Protein	25g
Total Fat	15g
Sugars	5g
Carbs	10g
Fiber	3g
Vitamin C	60mg

Practical Tips:

Soak wooden skewers in water for 30 minutes before grilling to prevent burning.

Preparation Time: 20 minutes

27. Quinoa and Black Bean Stuffed Peppers

Ingredients:

2 bell peppers, halved and seeds removed

1/2 cup cooked quinoa

1/2 cup canned black beans, rinsed and drained

1/4 cup corn kernels

1/4 cup diced tomatoes

1/4 cup shredded cheddar cheese

1 tablespoon chopped cilantro

1 teaspoon chili powder

Salt and pepper to taste

Preparation:

Preheat oven to 375°F.

In a bowl, mix cooked quinoa, black beans, corn, diced tomatoes, cheddar cheese, cilantro, chili powder, salt, and pepper.

Fill each bell pepper half with the quinoa mixture.

Place stuffed peppers in a baking dish.

Cover with aluminum foil and bake for 25-30 minutes, until peppers are tender.

Serve hot. Preparation Time: 40 minutes

Nutrition Facts:

Nutrient	Amount
Calories	280
Protein	12g
Total Fat	8g
Sugars	5g
Carbs	40g
Fiber	10g
Vitamin A	4000 IU

Practical Tips:

Customize filling with your favorite vegetables and spices.

28. Salmon and Avocado Salad

Ingredients:

4oz grilled salmon fillet, flaked

1/2 avocado, sliced

2 cups mixed greens

1/4 cup cherry tomatoes, halved

1/4 cup cucumber, sliced

1 tablespoon olive oil

1 tablespoon balsamic vinegar

Salt and pepper to taste

Preparation:

In a large bowl, combine mixed greens, cherry tomatoes, cucumber, and grilled salmon.

Drizzle with olive oil and balsamic vinegar.

Season with salt and pepper.

Top with sliced avocado.

Serve immediately.

Nutrition Facts:

Use leftover grilled salmon for an easy meal.

Preparation Time: 15 minutes

Nutrient	Amount
Calories	320
Protein	20g
Total Fat	22g
Sugars	4g
Carbs	15g
Fiber	8g
Vitamin D	400 IU

29. Eggplant and Tomato Bake

Ingredients:

1 large eggplant, sliced

2 tomatoes, sliced

1/4 cup grated Parmesan cheese

2 tablespoons olive oil

1 tablespoon balsamic vinegar

2 cloves garlic, minced

1 teaspoon dried basil

Salt and pepper to taste

Preparation:

Preheat oven to 375°F.

Arrange eggplant slices on a baking sheet lined with parchment paper.

In a small bowl, mix olive oil, balsamic vinegar, minced garlic, dried basil, salt, and pepper.

Brush the eggplant slices with the olive oil mixture.

Top each eggplant slice with a slice of tomato.

Sprinkle grated Parmesan cheese over the tomatoes.

Bake for 20-25 minutes, until eggplant is tender and cheese is golden brown

Serve hot as a side dish or over cooked quinoa or brown rice.

Nutrition Facts:

Nutrient	Amount
Calories	220
Protein	7g
Total Fat	14g
Sugars	7g
Carbs	18g
Fiber	8g
Vitamin C	15mg

30. Turkey and Vegetable Lettuce Wraps

Ingredients:

6 oz ground turkey

1/2 cup diced bell peppers

1/4 cup diced onion

1/4 cup diced tomatoes

1/4 cup shredded carrots

1 tablespoon olive oil

1 tablespoon soy sauce

1 tablespoon hoisin sauce

1 teaspoon sesame oil

1 teaspoon minced garlic

Butter lettuce leaves

Preparation:

Heat olive oil in a skillet over medium heat.

Add minced garlic and cook until fragrant, about 1 minute.

Add ground turkey and cook until browned.

Add diced bell peppers, onion, tomatoes, and shredded carrots. Cook until vegetables are tender.

Stir in soy sauce, hoisin sauce, and sesame oil. Cook for an additional 2 minutes.

Spoon the turkey and vegetable mixture into butter lettuce leaves.

Nutrition Facts:

Nutrient	Amount
Calories	280
Protein	20g
Total Fat	15g
Sugars	5g
Carbs	15g
Fiber	5g
Iron	3mg

31. Chickpea Salad

Ingredients:

1 can (15 oz) chickpeas, drained and rinsed

1/2 cucumber, diced

1/2 bell pepper, diced

1/4 red onion, finely chopped

2 tablespoons chopped fresh parsley

2 tablespoons olive oil

1 tablespoon lemon juice

Salt and pepper to taste

Preparation:

In a large bowl, combine chickpeas, cucumber, bell pepper, red onion, and parsley.

Drizzle olive oil and lemon juice over the salad.

Season with salt and pepper to taste.

Toss gently to combine.

Serve chilled or at room temperature.

Nutrition Facts:

Nutrient	Amount
Calories	280
Protein	10g
Total Fat	10g
Sugars	4g
Carbs	35g
Fiber	10g
Vitamin K	30mcg

Practical Tips:

Add feta cheese or olives for extra flavor. Preparation Time: 10 minutes

32. Tofu Stir-Fry with Vegetables

Ingredients:

6 oz firm tofu, cubed

1 cup broccoli florets

1/2 bell pepper, sliced

1/2 carrot, sliced

1/4 cup sliced mushrooms

2 tablespoons soy sauce

1 tablespoon hoisin sauce

1 tablespoon olive oil

1 teaspoon minced ginger

1 clove garlic, minced

Cooked brown rice for serving

Preparation:

Heat olive oil in a large skillet over medium heat.

Add minced garlic and ginger, and cook for 1 minute.

Add tofu cubes and cook until golden brown on all sides.

Add broccoli, bell pepper, carrot, and mushrooms to the skillet.

Stir in soy sauce and hoisin sauce.

Cook for 5-7 minutes until vegetables are tender and tofu is heated through.

Serve over cooked brown rice.

Nutrition Facts:

Nutrient	Amount
Calories	320
Protein	18g
Total Fat	15g
Sugars	5g
Carbs	35g
Fiber	8g
Iron	3mg

Practical Tips:

Use pre-cut vegetables for a quicker preparation. Preparation Time: 20 minutes

33. Caprese Salad Skewers

Ingredients:

12 cherry tomatoes

12 small fresh mozzarella balls (bocconcini)

12 fresh basil leaves

2 tablespoons balsamic glaze

Salt and pepper to taste

Preparation:

Thread one cherry tomato, one mozzarella ball, and one basil leaf onto each skewer.

Arrange skewers on a serving platter.

Drizzle balsamic glaze over the skewers.

Season with salt and pepper to taste.

Serve immediately.

Nutrition Facts:

Nutrient	Amount
Calories	160
Protein	8g
Total Fat	10g
Sugars	3g
Carbs	8g
Fiber	1g
Vitamin A	300 IU

Practical Tips:

Use wooden skewers for serving.

Preparation Time: 10 minutes

34. Spinach and Mushroom Omelette

Ingredients:

2 large eggs

1/2 cup fresh spinach leaves

1/4 cup sliced mushrooms

2 tablespoons shredded cheese (cheddar or mozzarella)

1 tablespoon olive oil

Salt and pepper to taste

Preparation:

In a small bowl, beat the eggs until well combined.

Heat olive oil in a non-stick skillet over medium heat.

Add spinach leaves and sliced mushrooms to the skillet.

Cook until spinach is wilted and mushrooms are tender.

Pour beaten eggs over the vegetables in the skillet.

Sprinkle shredded cheese over the eggs.

Cook until the edges are set and the bottom is golden brown.

Carefully fold the omelette in half with a spatula.

Cook for another minute until the cheese is melted and the eggs are cooked through.

Season with salt and pepper to taste.

Serve hot.

Nutrition Facts:

Nutrient	Amount
Calories	280
Protein	18g
Total Fat	20g
Sugars	2g
Carbs	4g
Fiber	2g
Vitamin D	2.5mcg

Practical Tips:

Customize with your favorite vegetables and cheese. Preparation Time: 10 minutes

35. Grilled Shrimp Skewers with Pineapple

Ingredients:

8oz large shrimp, peeled and deveined

1 cup pineapple chunks

1/4 cup soy sauce

2 tablespoons honey

1 tablespoon olive oil

1 teaspoon minced garlic

Wooden skewers, soaked in water

Preparation:

In a bowl, whisk together soy sauce, honey, olive oil, and minced garlic.

Thread shrimp and pineapple alternately onto skewers.

Place skewers in a shallow dish and pour marinade over them.

Cover and refrigerate for at least 30 minutes.

Preheat grill to medium-high heat.

Remove skewers from marinade and discard excess marinade.

Grill skewers for 2-3 minutes on each side, until shrimp is cooked through and pineapple is caramelized.

Nutrition Facts:

Nutrient	Amount
Calories	240
Protein	20g
Total Fat	8g
Sugars	18g
Carbs	25g
Fiber	2g
Vitamin C	30mg

Practical Tips:

Serve with a side of steamed vegetables or quinoa. Preparation Time: 20 minutes

36. Turkey and Veggie Lettuce Wraps

Ingredients:

6oz ground turkey

1/2 cup diced bell peppers

1/2 cup diced zucchini

1/4 cup diced onion

2 cloves garlic, minced

2 tablespoons soy sauce

1 tablespoon olive oil

Butter lettuce leaves

Preparation:

Heat olive oil in a skillet over medium heat.

Add minced garlic and cook until fragrant.

Add ground turkey and cook until browned.

Add diced bell peppers, zucchini, and onion. Cook until vegetables are tender.

Stir in soy sauce and cook for another 2-3 minutes.

Spoon the turkey and vegetable mixture into butter lettuce leaves.

Serve immediately.

Nutrition Facts:

Nutrient	Amount
Calories	250
Protein	20g
Total Fat	12g
Sugars	4g
Carbs	15g
Fiber	4g
Iron	3mg

Practical Tips:

Top with chopped green onions or cilantro for extra flavor.

Preparation Time: 20 minutes

37. Mediterranean Chickpea Salad

Ingredients:

1 can (15 oz) chickpeas, drained and rinsed

1/2 cucumber, diced

1/2 bell pepper, diced

1/4 red onion, finely chopped

1/4 cup Kalamata olives, sliced

2 tablespoons chopped fresh parsley

2 tablespoons olive oil

1 tablespoon lemon juice

Salt and pepper to taste

Preparation:

In a large bowl, combine chickpeas, cucumber, bell pepper, red onion, olives, and parsley.

Drizzle olive oil and lemon juice over the salad.

Season with salt and pepper to taste.

Toss gently to combine.

Serve chilled or at room temperature.

Nutrition Facts:

Nutrient	Amount
Calories	280
Protein	10g
Total Fat	12g
Sugars	5g
Carbs	35g
Fiber	10g
Vitamin C	30mg

Practical Tips:

Add crumbled feta cheese for extra creaminess.

Preparation Time: 15 minutes

38. Grilled Salmon with Asparagus

Ingredients:

6oz salmon fillet

1 bunch asparagus, trimmed

1 tablespoon olive oil

1 teaspoon lemon zest

1 tablespoon lemon juice

Salt and pepper to taste

Preparation:

Preheat grill to medium-high heat.

Brush salmon fillet and asparagus spears with olive oil.

Season with lemon zest, lemon juice, salt, and pepper.

Place salmon fillet and asparagus spears on the grill.

Grill for 4-5 minutes per side, or until salmon is cooked through and asparagus is tender.

Serve hot.

Nutrition Facts:

Nutrient	Amount
Calories	300
Protein	25g
Total Fat	18g
Sugars	3g
Carbs	10g
Fiber	5g
Vitamin D	500 IU

Practical Tips:

Serve with a squeeze of fresh lemon juice.

Preparation Time: 15 minutes

39. Egg and Vegetable Muffin Cups

Ingredients:

4 eggs

1/2 cup diced bell peppers

1/4 cup diced onion

1/4 cup chopped spinach

1/4 cup shredded cheese (cheddar or mozzarella)

Salt and pepper to taste

Preparation:

Preheat oven to 350°F.

In a bowl, whisk together eggs, diced bell peppers, onion, chopped spinach, shredded cheese, salt, and pepper.

Divide the egg mixture evenly among muffin cups.

Bake for 20-25 minutes, or until the muffin cups are set and lightly golden.

Allow to cool slightly before serving.

Nutrition Facts:

Nutrient	Amount
Calories	180
Protein	12g
Total Fat	10g
Sugars	3g
Carbs	10g
Fiber	2g
Vitamin A	500 IU

Practical Tips:

Use silicone muffin liners for easy removal.

Preparation Time: 30 minutes

40. Greek Yogurt Berry Smoothie

Ingredients:

1/2 cup Greek yogurt

1/2 cup mixed berries (strawberries, blueberries, raspberries)

1/2 banana

1/2 cup almond milk (unsweetened)

1 tablespoon honey (optional)

Ice cubes

Preparation:

Place Greek yogurt, mixed berries, banana, almond milk, honey, and ice cubes in a blender.

Blend until smooth and creamy.

Pour into glasses and serve immediately.

Nutrition Facts:

Nutrient	Amount
Calories	180
Protein	10g
Total Fat	3g
Sugars	15g
Carbs	25g
Fiber	5g
Vitamin C	20mg

Practical Tips:

Add a scoop of protein powder for extra protein.

Preparation Time: 5 minutes

41. Mediterranean Grilled Chicken Salad

Ingredients:

6oz chicken breast, grilled and sliced

2 cups mixed greens

1/2 cup cherry tomatoes, halved

1/4 cup cucumber, sliced

1/4 cup Kalamata olives, pitted

2 tablespoons crumbled feta cheese

1 tablespoon olive oil

1 tablespoon balsamic vinegar

1 teaspoon dried oregano

Salt and pepper to taste

Preparation:

In a large bowl, combine mixed greens, cherry tomatoes, cucumber, and Kalamata olives.

Top with grilled chicken slices and crumbled feta cheese.

In a small bowl, whisk together olive oil, balsamic vinegar, dried oregano, salt, and pepper.

Drizzle the dressing over the salad.

Toss gently to combine.

Nutrition Facts:

Nutrient	Amount
Calories	320
Protein	25g
Total Fat	18g
Sugars	5g
Carbs	15g
Fiber	5g
Vitamin A	4000 IU

Practical Tips:

Add a squeeze of lemon juice for extra freshness. Preparation Time: 20 minutes

42. Greek Quinoa Salad

Ingredients:

1 cup cooked quinoa
1/2 cucumber, diced
1/2 bell pepper, diced
1/4 cup diced red onion
1/4 cup cherry tomatoes, halved
1/4 cup crumbled feta cheese
2 tablespoons chopped fresh parsley
2 tablespoons olive oil
1 tablespoon lemon juice
1 teaspoon dried oregano
Salt and pepper to taste

Preparation:

In a large bowl, combine cooked quinoa, cucumber, bell pepper, red onion, cherry tomatoes, feta cheese, and parsley.
In a small bowl, whisk together olive oil, lemon juice, dried oregano, salt, and pepper.
Pour the dressing over the quinoa salad.
Toss gently to combine.
Serve chilled or at room temperature.

Nutrition Facts:

Nutrient	Amount
Calories	280
Protein	8g
Total Fat	15g
Sugars	5g
Carbs	30g
Fiber	5g
Iron	3mg

Practical Tips:

Add chopped olives for extra flavor. Preparation Time: 15 minutes

43. Mediterranean Stuffed Bell Peppers

Ingredients:

2 bell peppers, halved and seeds removed

1/2 cup cooked quinoa

1/2 cup canned chickpeas, rinsed and drained

1/4 cup diced tomatoes

1/4 cup diced cucumber

2 tablespoons chopped fresh parsley

2 tablespoons crumbled feta cheese

1 tablespoon olive oil

1 tablespoon lemon juice

1 teaspoon dried oregano

Salt and pepper to taste

Preparation:

Preheat oven to 375°F.

In a large bowl, combine cooked quinoa, chickpeas, diced tomatoes, diced cucumber, parsley, and feta cheese.

In a small bowl, whisk together olive oil, lemon juice, dried oregano, salt, and pepper.

Pour the dressing over the quinoa mixture and toss to combine.

Spoon the quinoa mixture into each bell pepper half.

Place stuffed bell peppers in a baking dish.

Cover with aluminum foil and bake for 25-30 minutes, until peppers are tender.

Serve hot.

Nutrition Facts:

Nutrient	Amount
Calories	280
Protein	10g
Total Fat	12g
Sugars	5g
Carbs	35g
Fiber	10g
Vitamin C	60mg

44. Mediterranean Baked Salmon

Ingredients:

6oz salmon fillet

1/4 cup diced tomatoes

2 tablespoons sliced Kalamata olives

1 tablespoon capers

1 tablespoon chopped fresh parsley

1 tablespoon olive oil

1 teaspoon minced garlic

1/2 teaspoon dried oregano

Salt and pepper to taste

Lemon wedges for serving

Preparation:

Preheat oven to 375°F.

Place salmon fillet on a baking sheet lined with parchment paper.

In a small bowl, mix together diced tomatoes, sliced olives, capers, parsley, olive oil, minced garlic, dried oregano, salt, and pepper.

Spoon the tomato mixture over the salmon fillet.

Bake for 15-20 minutes, or until salmon is cooked through and flakes easily with a fork.

Serve hot with lemon wedges.

Nutrition Facts:

Nutrient	Amount
Calories	320
Protein	25g
Total Fat	20g
Sugars	2g
Carbs	5g
Fiber	2g
Vitamin D	400 IU

Practical Tips: Serve with a side of roasted vegetables or quinoa.

45. Greek Yogurt Parfait with Honey and Almonds

Ingredients:

1/2 cup Greek yogurt

1/4 cup mixed berries (strawberries, blueberries, raspberries)

1 tablespoon honey

2 tablespoons sliced almonds

Preparation:

In a serving glass or bowl, layer Greek yogurt, mixed berries, honey, and sliced almonds.

Repeat layers until ingredients are used up.

Serve immediately.

Nutrition Facts:

Nutrient	Amount
Calories	220
Protein	15g
Total Fat	10g
Sugars	20g
Carbs	25g
Fiber	5g
Calcium	200mg

Practical Tips:

Use plain Greek yogurt for a tangy flavor.

Preparation Time: 5 minutes

46. Spinach and Feta Egg Muffins

Ingredients:

4 large eggs

1 cup baby spinach, chopped

1/4 cup crumbled feta cheese

1/4 cup diced red bell pepper

Salt and pepper to taste

Preparation:

Preheat oven to 350°F (175°C) and grease a muffin tin.

In a mixing bowl, whisk together eggs, chopped spinach, feta cheese, diced red bell pepper, salt, and pepper.

Pour the egg mixture evenly into the muffin tin.

Bake for 20-25 minutes or until the egg muffins are set and lightly golden.

Allow to cool slightly before serving.

Nutrition Facts:

Nutrient	Amount
Calories	120
Protein	9g
Total Fat	7g
Sugars	1g
Carbs	4g
Fiber	1g
Vitamin A	1500 IU

Practical Tips:

These egg muffins can be stored in the refrigerator for up to 3 days.

Preparation Time: 30 minutes

47. Mediterranean Tuna Salad

Ingredients:

1 can (5 oz) tuna in water, drained

1/4 cup diced cucumber

1/4 cup diced tomato

2 tablespoons chopped red onion

2 tablespoons sliced Kalamata olives

1 tablespoon chopped fresh parsley

1 tablespoon olive oil

1 tablespoon lemon juice

Salt and pepper to taste

Preparation:

In a mixing bowl, combine drained tuna, diced cucumber, diced tomato, chopped red onion,

sliced Kalamata olives, and chopped fresh parsley.

Drizzle olive oil and lemon juice over the salad.

Season with salt and pepper to taste.

Toss gently to combine.

Serve chilled.

Nutrition Facts:

Nutrient	Amount
Calories	180
Protein	20g
Total Fat	9g
Sugars	2g
Carbs	4g
Fiber	2g
Iron	2.5mg

Practical Tips:

Serve the tuna salad on a bed of mixed greens for a heartier meal.
Preparation Time: 10 minutes

48. Greek Chicken Skewers with Tzatziki Sauce

Ingredients:

6oz chicken breast, cut into cubes

1/4 cup Greek yogurt

1 tablespoon olive oil

1 tablespoon lemon juice

1 teaspoon minced garlic

1 teaspoon dried oregano

Salt and pepper to taste

Tzatziki sauce for serving

Preparation:

In a mixing bowl, combine Greek yogurt, olive oil, lemon juice, minced garlic, dried oregano, salt, and pepper.

Add chicken cubes to the marinade and toss to coat. Marinate for at least 30 minutes.

Thread the marinated chicken cubes onto skewers.

Preheat grill or grill pan over medium-high heat.

Grill the chicken skewers for 5-7 minutes on each side or until cooked through.

Serve hot with tzatziki sauce for dipping.

Nutrition Facts:

Nutrient	Amount
Calories	250
Protein	30g
Total Fat	12g
Sugars	2g
Carbs	4g
Fiber	1g
Calcium	100mg

Practical Tips:

Soak wooden skewers in water for 30 minutes before grilling to prevent burning.
Preparation Time: 40 minutes (including marinating time)

49. Mediterranean Lentil Soup

Ingredients:

1 cup dried green lentils

4 cups vegetable broth

1/2 cup diced carrots

1/2 cup diced celery

1/2 cup diced onion

2 cloves garlic, minced

1 teaspoon dried thyme

1 teaspoon dried oregano

Salt and pepper to taste

Fresh parsley for garnish

Preparation:

Rinse the dried green lentils under cold water and drain.

In a large pot, combine rinsed lentils, vegetable broth, diced carrots, diced celery, diced onion, minced garlic, dried thyme, and dried oregano.

Bring the soup to a boil, then reduce heat to low and simmer for 25-30 minutes or until lentils and vegetables are tender.

Season with salt and pepper to taste.

Ladle the soup into bowls and garnish with fresh parsley before serving.

Nutrition Facts:

Nutrient	Amount
Calories	200
Protein	15g
Total Fat	1g
Sugars	3g
Carbs	35g
Fiber	15g
Iron	4mg

Practical Tips:

Add a squeeze of lemon juice before serving for extra brightness.

Preparation Time: 45 minutes

50. Mediterranean Chicken and Veggie Skewers

Ingredients:

6 oz chicken breast, cut into cubes

1/2 cup cherry tomatoes

1/2 cup zucchini, sliced

1/2 cup bell peppers, diced

1/4 cup red onion, diced

2 tablespoons olive oil

2 cloves garlic, minced

1 teaspoon dried oregano

1 teaspoon dried thyme

Salt and pepper to taste

Lemon wedges for serving

Preparation:

In a bowl, combine chicken cubes, cherry tomatoes, zucchini slices, diced bell peppers, and diced red onion.

In a separate small bowl, whisk together olive oil, minced garlic, dried oregano, dried thyme, salt, and pepper.

Pour the marinade over the chicken and vegetable mixture. Toss until everything is evenly coated. Let marinate for at least 30 minutes.

Preheat grill or grill pan over medium-high heat.

Thread the marinated chicken and vegetables onto skewers.

Grill the skewers for 4-5 minutes on each side, or until the chicken is cooked through and the vegetables are tender.

Nutrition Facts:

Nutrient	Amount
Calories	280
Protein	25g
Total Fat	15g
Sugars	5g
Carbs	10g
Fiber	3g
Vitamin C	40mg

This table provides a concise overview of intermittent fasting for beginners, covering key concepts, methods, health benefits, practical tips, and potential considerations.

Aspect	Description
What is Intermittent Fasting?	Intermittent fasting is an eating pattern that cycles between periods of fasting and eating.
Key Principles	- Fasting Periods: Restricting food intake for a set period. - Eating Windows: Consuming meals within specific time frames.
Health Benefits	- Weight Loss: Promotes fat loss and preserves muscle mass. - Improved Metabolic Health: Regulates blood sugar levels, insulin sensitivity, and cholesterol levels. - Enhanced Brain Function: Supports cognitive function and may reduce the risk of neurodegenerative diseases.
Common Fasting Methods	- 16/8 Method: Fasting for 16 hours and eating within an 8-hour window. - 5:2 Diet: Eating normally for 5 days and restricting calorie intake for 2 non-consecutive days. - Alternate Day Fasting: Alternating between fasting days and eating days.
Getting Started	- Choose a fasting method that aligns with your lifestyle and preferences. - Start gradually by gradually increasing fasting periods and adjusting meal timings.
Nutrition Guidelines	- Focus on whole, nutrient-dense foods during eating windows. - Stay hydrated and drink plenty of water during fasting periods.
Exercise Recommendations	- Incorporate regular physical activity into your routine, aiming for a mix of cardio, strength training, and flexibility exercises. - Consider timing workouts during eating windows for optimal performance and recovery.
Mindset and Motivation	- Adopt a positive mindset and view intermittent fasting as a sustainable lifestyle change rather than a quick fix. - Stay motivated by setting realistic goals, tracking progress, and celebrating achievements.
Potential Risks	- Nutrient Deficiencies: Ensure adequate nutrient intake during eating windows to prevent deficiencies. - Disordered Eating: Monitor for signs of disordered eating behaviors and seek support if needed. - Medical Conditions: Consult with a healthcare professional before starting intermittent fasting, especially if you have underlying medical conditions.
Resources and Support	- Seek reliable information from reputable sources, books, and scientific studies. - Join online communities or support groups to connect with others following intermittent fasting and share experiences and tips.

Here's the 28-day meal plan with each day broken down

Week 1:

Day 1:
Breakfast: Egg and Vegetable Breakfast Muffins
Lunch: Avocado and Shrimp Salad
Dinner: Spinach and Feta Stuffed Chicken Breast
Snack: Greek Yogurt and Berry Parfait

Day 2:
Breakfast: Greek Yogurt Parfait with Honey and Almonds
Lunch: Chickpea and Tomato Salad
Dinner: Quinoa and Vegetable Stir-Fry
Snack: Lentil and Vegetable Soup

Day 3:
Breakfast: Spinach and Feta Egg Muffins
Lunch: Mediterranean Tuna Salad
Dinner: Grilled Salmon with Asparagus
Snack: Mediterranean Lentil Soup

Day 4:
Breakfast: Greek Yogurt Berry Smoothie
Lunch: Tofu Stir-Fry with Vegetables
Dinner: Turkey and Spinach Stuffed Bell Peppers
Snack: Mediterranean Chickpea Salad

Day 5:
Breakfast: Egg and Vegetable Muffin Cups
Lunch: Mediterranean Grilled Chicken Salad
Dinner: Eggplant and Tomato Bake
Snack: Greek Yogurt Parfait with Honey and Almonds

Day 6:
Breakfast: Greek Quinoa Salad
Lunch: Mediterranean Baked Salmon
Dinner: Turkey and Vegetable Skewers
Snack: Greek Yogurt Parfait with Honey and Almonds

Day 7:
Breakfast: Mediterranean Stuffed Bell Peppers
Lunch: Mediterranean Chickpea Bowl
Dinner: Grilled Chicken and Quinoa Salad
Snack: Spinach and Feta Egg Muffins

Week 2:

Day 8:
Breakfast: Greek Yogurt and Berry Parfait
Lunch: Spinach and Feta Stuffed Chicken Breast
Dinner: Quinoa and Vegetable Stir-Fry
Snack: Avocado and Egg Salad

Continue this pattern for the remaining days, alternating between the provided recipes and ensuring a balanced mix of protein, carbohydrates, and healthy fats for each meal

General Considerations and Advice for Starting Intermittent Fasting

Congratulations on taking the first step towards exploring intermittent fasting! As you embark on this journey, it's important to approach it with a mindset of curiosity, openness, and self-compassion. Here are some general considerations and advice to guide you along the way:

Start Slowly: Intermittent fasting is not a one-size-fits-all approach, and it's essential to find a fasting schedule that works for you. Consider starting with shorter fasting periods, such as a 12-hour overnight fast, and gradually increasing the duration as you become more comfortable.

Listen to Your Body: Pay attention to your body's hunger cues and energy levels. If you feel overly fatigued or lightheaded during fasting periods, it may be a sign that you need to adjust your fasting schedule or consider incorporating more nutrient-dense foods into your meals.

Stay Hydrated: Proper hydration is key to supporting your body during fasting periods. Be sure to drink plenty of water throughout the day, especially during fasting periods, to help curb hunger and maintain energy levels.

Focus on Nutrient-Dense Foods: When breaking your fast, prioritize nutrient-dense foods such as fruits, vegetables, lean proteins, whole grains, and healthy fats. These foods will provide your body with the essential nutrients it needs to thrive and support overall health.

Be Patient and Persistent: Rome wasn't built in a day, and neither are the benefits of intermittent fasting. Give yourself time to adapt to this new eating pattern, and don't be discouraged by setbacks or challenges along the way. Consistency and persistence are key to long-term success.

Seek Support: Consider joining online communities, forums, or support groups where you can connect with others who are also exploring intermittent fasting. Sharing experiences, tips, and encouragement can provide valuable support and motivation on your journey.

Consult with a Healthcare Professional: Before starting any new diet or lifestyle regimen, especially if you have underlying health conditions or concerns, it's important to consult with a healthcare professional. They can provide personalized guidance based on your individual needs and help ensure that intermittent fasting is safe and appropriate for you

Remember, intermittent fasting is not about deprivation or punishment—it's about nourishing your body, supporting your health, and finding a sustainable approach to eating that works for you. Be kind to yourself, embrace the journey, and celebrate the progress you make along the way. Here's to a healthier, happier you

BOOK 2

Anti-inflammatory Diet Cookbook for Beginners

Anti-inflammatory Diet Cookbook for Beginners

"Embrace a Lifestyle of Anti-Inflammation: Rediscover Wellness through Inner Healing and Liberation from Chronic Inflammation!"

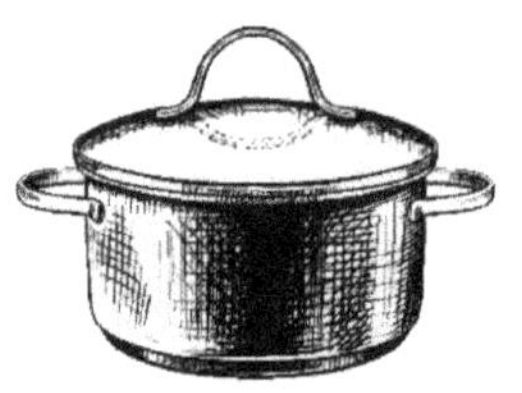

Lisa Howell

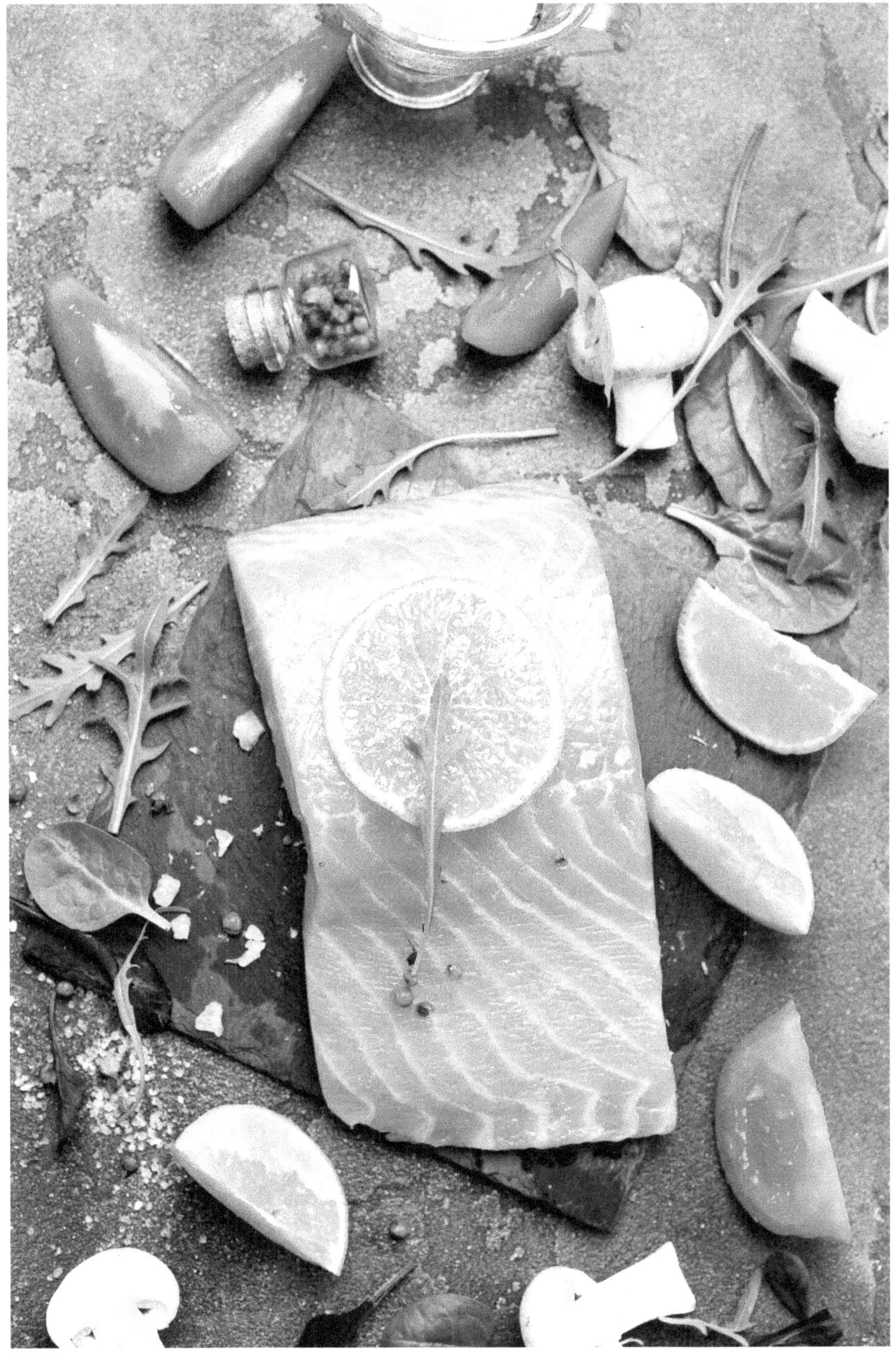

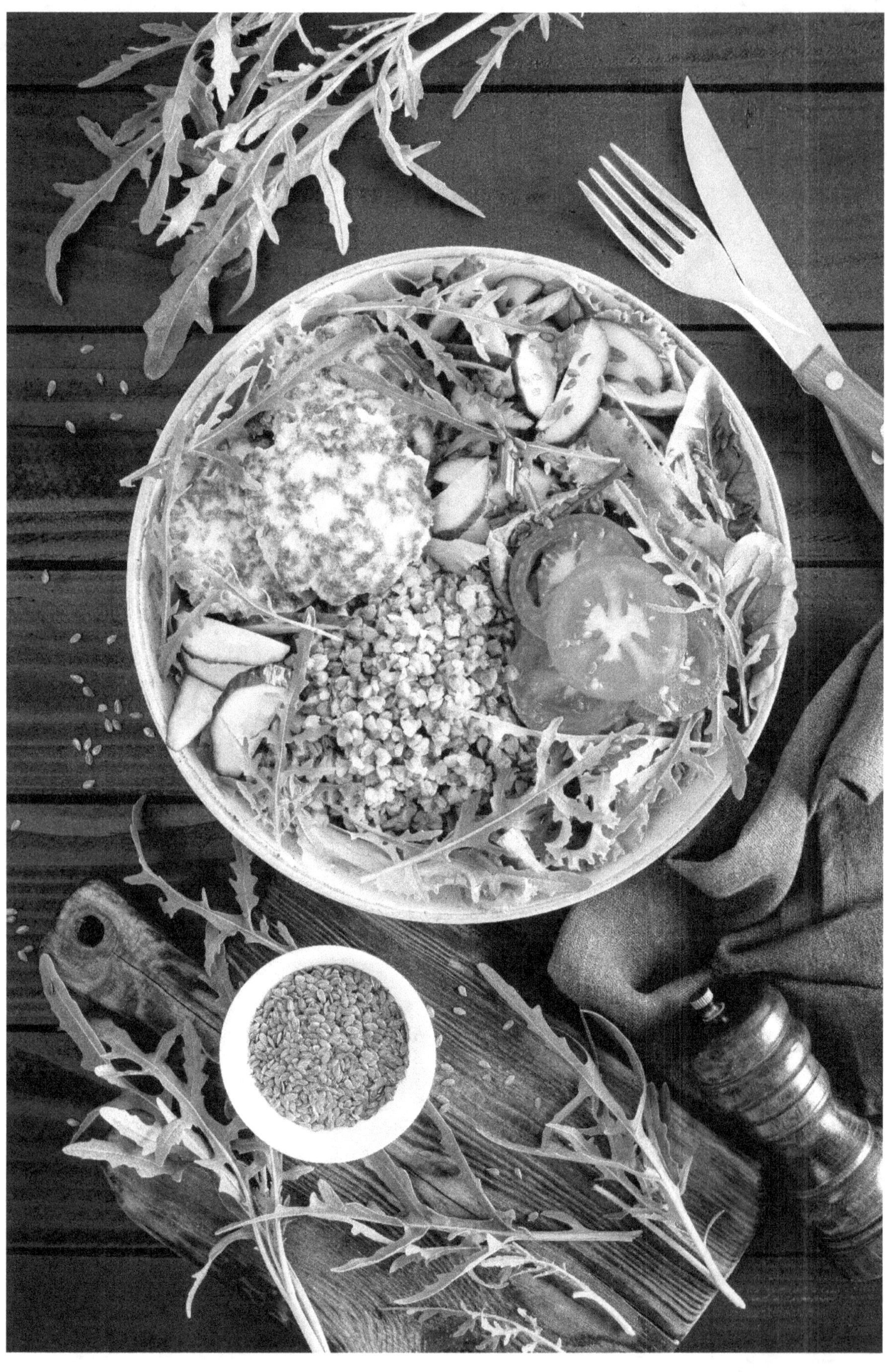

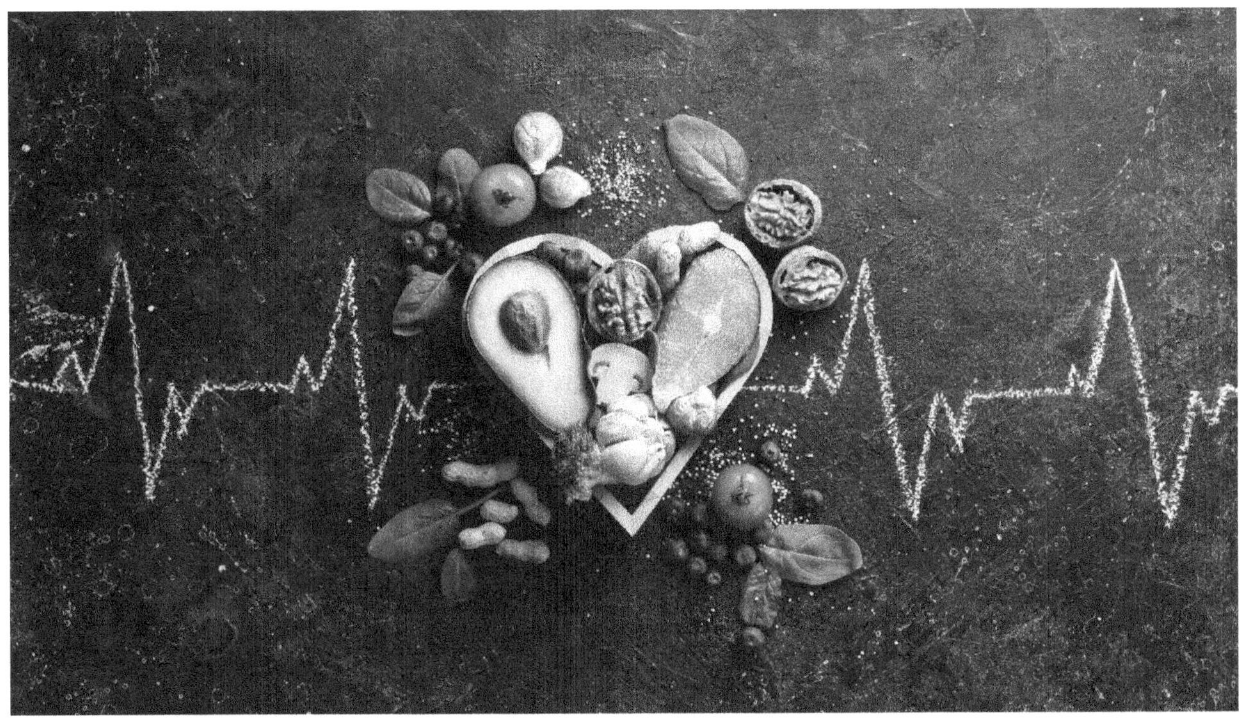

Welcome to "The Ultimate Anti-Inflammatory Diet: Your Pathway to Optimal Health." In these pages, you will embark on a transformative journey towards vibrant well-being and discover the incredible power of nutrition to heal and restore your body.

Introduction

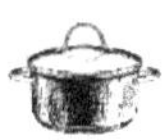

In today's fast-paced and hectic world, prioritizing our health has become more important than ever. One way to promote overall well-being is by adopting an anti-inflammatory diet. This approach focuses on consuming foods that help reduce inflammation in the body, leading to numerous benefits for our health and vitality. So why should you consider pursuing an anti-inflammatory diet? Let's explore the advantages and disadvantages.

Advantages of an Anti-Inflammatory Diet:

1. Reduced Inflammation: Chronic inflammation has been linked to various health issues, including heart disease, arthritis, and autoimmune disorders. By following an anti-inflammatory diet, you can help reduce inflammation in the body, potentially preventing or managing these conditions.

2. Enhanced Immune Function: A healthy immune system is vital for warding off illnesses and infections. The nutrients found in an anti-inflammatory diet, such as antioxidants, vitamins, and minerals, can support a robust immune response and keep your body strong.

3. Weight Management: Excess weight can contribute to inflammation and increase the risk of chronic diseases. An anti-inflammatory diet promotes whole, nutrient-dense foods and emphasizes portion control, making it easier to maintain a healthy weight.

4. Improved Digestive Health: Many gastrointestinal issues, such as bloating, gas, and irritable bowel syndrome (IBS), are associated with inflammation. By incorporating anti-inflammatory foods and avoiding triggers, you can help soothe your digestive system and promote optimal gut health.

5. Balanced Blood Sugar Levels: Unstable blood sugar levels can lead to inflammation and increase the risk of conditions like diabetes. An anti-inflammatory diet, rich in fiber and low in refined sugars, can help stabilize blood sugar levels, supporting overall metabolic health.

Disadvantages of an Anti-Inflammatory Diet:

1. Individual Variations: While an anti-inflammatory diet can benefit most individuals, there may be variations in how our bodies respond to specific foods. It's essential to listen to your body and make adjustments based on your unique needs and sensitivities.

2. Dietary Restriction: Some individuals may find it challenging to adapt to the dietary changes required for an anti-inflammatory diet, especially if they have specific dietary preferences or restrictions. However, with proper planning and creativity, a wide range of delicious and nutritious options can still be enjoyed.

Preventive Medical Examinations:

Regular medical check-ups are crucial for maintaining optimal health. Alongside adopting an anti-inflammatory diet, it's advisable to undergo preventive medical examinations recommended by healthcare professionals. These may include routine blood tests, cholesterol checks, blood pressure monitoring, and screenings for conditions like diabetes and certain cancers.

Symptoms of Inflammation:

Inflammation can manifest in various ways throughout the body. Common symptoms include persistent fatigue, joint pain or stiffness, frequent infections, digestive issues, skin problems, and mood changes. If you experience these symptoms or suspect chronic inflammation, it's important to consult with a healthcare provider for proper evaluation and guidance.

Causes of Inflammation:

Inflammation can be triggered by various factors, including poor diet, sedentary lifestyle, chronic stress, environmental toxins, and certain medical conditions. Adopting an anti-inflammatory diet, along with lifestyle modifications, can address some of these underlying causes and help manage inflammation effectively.

Remember, embarking on an anti-inflammatory diet is a journey towards improved health and well-being. It's important to approach it with a relaxed and pleasant mindset. Listen to your body, make gradual changes, and seek guidance from healthcare professionals or nutrition experts as needed. By incorporating an anti-inflammatory diet into your lifestyle, you can take proactive steps towards nurturing your body and enjoying a vibrant, inflammation-free life.

A Mindset for Long-Term Success: Embracing the Joy of Healthy Eating and Cooking

Embarking on a journey to change our way of eating and cooking can feel overwhelming at times. However, by cultivating the right mindset, we can set ourselves up for long-term success and effortlessly maintain a healthy regimen. Let's explore a mindset that embraces the joy of healthy eating, approaches an anti-inflammatory diet with ease, and allows healthy habits to become second nature, all in a relaxed and psychoanalytic tone.

1. Nurture a Positive Relationship with Food: Instead of viewing food as the enemy or restricting ourselves, let's foster a positive and nurturing relationship with the food we consume. Recognize that food is nourishment for both the body and the soul. Approach mealtime as an opportunity to savor and enjoy the flavors, textures, and colors that nature provides.

2. Embrace Mindful Eating: Mindful eating is a powerful practice that involves being fully present and aware of each bite we take. Slow down, savor each mouthful, and pay attention to the sensations, tastes, and aromas. By doing so, we can cultivate a deeper appreciation for the nourishment we receive and develop a greater understanding of our body's hunger and satiety cues.

3. Explore the Culinary Arts: Cooking can be a creative and therapeutic outlet. Embrace the joy of exploring new recipes, experimenting with different flavors, and trying out new cooking techniques. See the kitchen as your canvas and cooking as an opportunity for self-expression. Allow yourself to be inspired by fresh ingredients and cultural cuisines, and let your creativity flourish.

4. Embrace the Power of Preparation: Adopting an anti-inflammatory diet becomes easier when we prioritize preparation. Dedicate time to plan your meals, create a grocery list, and stock up on wholesome ingredients. Prepping meals in advance and having healthy snacks readily available can help eliminate decision fatigue and prevent impulsive, less healthy choices.

5. Cultivate Self-Compassion: Remember, change takes time, and it's important to be kind to ourselves along the way. Embrace the process and acknowledge that there may be ups and downs. Treat setbacks as learning opportunities rather than failures.

Celebrate small victories and milestones, and recognize that each step forward is a step towards improved well-being.

6. Find a Supportive Community: Surround yourself with like-minded individuals who share similar goals and aspirations. Connect with others who are also on a journey towards better health and engage in discussions, share recipes, and provide support. Having a community of individuals who understand and empathize with your experiences can be invaluable.

7. Embrace Flexibility: While it's important to have a general framework for an anti-inflammatory diet, it's equally important to embrace flexibility. Allow yourself to indulge in occasional treats or deviations from the plan without guilt. Strive for balance rather than perfection. Remember that sustainable change is built on a foundation of flexibility and self-compassion.

By adopting this mindset, we can approach an anti-inflammatory diet with joy and ease. We can transform healthy eating and cooking into habits that effortlessly support our overall well-being. So, let's embark on this journey with open hearts and minds, knowing that the choices we make today will shape our healthier, happier future selves.

Recommended Foods for an Anti-Inflammatory Diet

When it comes to following an anti-inflammatory diet, choosing the right foods can make a world of difference in your overall health and well-being. By incorporating nutrient-rich and anti-inflammatory foods into your daily meals, you can take proactive steps towards managing chronic health problems, increasing your energy levels, and reducing the need for medications. Let's explore some of the most recommended foods and create a shopping list to help you get started on your anti-inflammatory journey.

Fruits and Vegetables: Fill Your Plate with Color

Incorporating a variety of fruits and vegetables into your diet is essential. These vibrant gems are packed with essential vitamins, minerals, and antioxidants that help fight inflammation. Opt for colorful options like berries, cherries, oranges, spinach, kale, broccoli, and bell peppers. They not only add a burst of flavor to your meals but also provide numerous health benefits.

Whole Grains: Embrace Wholesome Choices

Replace refined grains with whole grains to maximize nutritional benefits. Whole grains like quinoa, brown rice, oats, and whole wheat bread are rich in fiber, vitamins, and minerals. They help regulate blood sugar levels, support digestion, and contribute to overall well-being.

Healthy Fats: Nourish Your Body

Include healthy fats in your diet to combat inflammation and provide energy. Avocados, nuts (such as almonds, walnuts, and cashews), seeds (such as flaxseeds and chia seeds), and olive oil are excellent sources of monounsaturated fats and omega-3 fatty acids. These fats have anti-inflammatory properties and promote heart health.

Fatty Fish: Dive into Omega-3 Goodness

Fatty fish like salmon, mackerel, and sardines are rich in omega-3 fatty acids. These healthy fats are known for their potent anti-inflammatory effects. Aim to include fatty fish in your meals at least twice a week to reap their benefits.

Legumes: Powerhouse of Plant-Based Protein

Legumes, including beans, lentils, chickpeas, and soy products like tofu, are excellent sources of plant-based protein. They are also packed with fiber, vitamins, and minerals. Incorporating legumes into your diet can help reduce inflammation and provide sustained energy throughout the day.

Herbs and Spices: Flavorful Health Boosters

Embrace the power of herbs and spices to enhance the taste and health benefits of your meals. Turmeric, ginger, garlic, cinnamon, and oregano are just a few examples of spices that have anti-inflammatory properties. Sprinkle them into your dishes or brew them into soothing teas for added flavor and health benefits.

Green Tea: Sip Your Way to Wellness Green tea is not only a refreshing beverage but also a potent anti-inflammatory elixir. Packed with antioxidants called catechins, green tea can help reduce inflammation and support overall health. Enjoy a cup or two throughout the day to reap its benefits.

Here are some additional foods that are beneficial for an anti-inflammatory diet:

Turmeric: Known for its powerful anti-inflammatory properties, turmeric contains curcumin, which helps reduce inflammation in the body. It can be used in various dishes or consumed as a supplement.

Ginger: Another spice with anti-inflammatory properties, ginger has been used for centuries to alleviate pain and reduce inflammation. It can be added to meals, brewed as a tea, or used in smoothies.

Berries: In addition to the mentioned assorted berries, include other varieties like raspberries, blackberries, and cranberries. They are rich in antioxidants and have anti-inflammatory effects.

Cherries: Apart from the mentioned cherries, tart cherries, specifically, have been found to possess potent anti-inflammatory properties. They can be consumed fresh, dried, or as cherry juice.

Pineapple: This tropical fruit contains bromelain, an enzyme that has anti-inflammatory effects. Enjoy fresh pineapple as a snack or add it to smoothies and salads.

Green leafy vegetables: Expand your leafy greens to include options like arugula, Swiss chard, and collard greens. These vegetables are packed with vitamins, minerals, and antioxidants that combat inflammation.

Sweet potatoes: Rich in antioxidants and fiber, sweet potatoes are a great addition to an anti-inflammatory diet. They can be baked, roasted, or mashed as a nutritious side dish.

Garlic: Adding flavor to your meals while offering anti-inflammatory benefits, garlic contains sulfur compounds that help reduce inflammation. Use it in cooking or enjoy it raw in dressings or sauces.

Dark chocolate: Opt for dark chocolate with a high cocoa content (70% or more) as it contains antioxidants that can help reduce inflammation. Enjoy a small piece as a treat.

Red grapes: Rich in resveratrol, a powerful antioxidant, red grapes have anti-inflammatory properties. Enjoy them as a snack or include them in salads and desserts.

Extra virgin olive oil: Use extra virgin olive oil as your primary cooking oil. It is rich in healthy monounsaturated fats and contains polyphenols that have anti-inflammatory effects. Remember to choose high-quality, organic, and minimally processed options whenever possible.

Extra Bonus

PRESSURE CANNING COOKBOOK

Lisa Howell

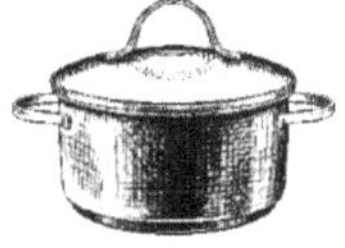

Explanation of the health benefits and impact on inflammation-related conditions and weight management

Setting the stage: Our bodies are incredible machines that work tirelessly to keep us healthy and balanced. However, sometimes they encounter challenges, such as injury or infection, that can lead to inflammation.

An empathetic approach: In this chapter, we will explore the fascinating world of inflammation, understand its effects on the body, and discover how we can support our well-being through the power of an anti-inflammatory diet.

Exploring Inflammation:

The body's natural defense: Inflammation is not your enemy; it is a vital response aimed at protecting and healing you. It's like a superhero swooping in to fight off invaders and repair damaged tissues.

The dual nature of inflammation: While acute inflammation is a temporary process that helps us heal, chronic inflammation can disrupt the delicate balance within our bodies and contribute to various health issues.

Unveiling the effects: Chronic inflammation has been linked to conditions like arthritis, autoimmune disorders, and digestive problems. Understanding these effects helps us appreciate the importance of managing inflammation effectively.

Losing weight can be a challenging journey, but with an anti-inflammatory diet, you can make positive changes that support your weight loss goals in a soothing and reassuring way. Here are some tips to help you along the way:

1. Emphasize Whole, Nutrient-Dense Foods: Focus on incorporating plenty of fresh fruits and vegetables, lean proteins, whole grains, and healthy fats into your meals. These foods provide essential nutrients while keeping you satisfied.

2. Include Anti-Inflammatory Foods: Choose foods with natural anti-inflammatory properties, such as fatty fish (salmon, mackerel), leafy greens (spinach, kale), berries,

turmeric, and ginger. These ingredients can help reduce inflammation in the body and support your weight loss efforts.

3. Mindful Eating: Practice mindful eating by paying attention to your body's hunger and fullness cues. Eat slowly, savor each bite, and listen to your body's signals to prevent overeating.

4. Portion Control: Be mindful of portion sizes and aim for balanced meals. Use smaller plates and bowls to help control portions visually. Include a variety of colorful vegetables to bulk up your meals without adding excessive calories.

5. Limit Processed Foods: Minimize or avoid processed foods high in added sugars, unhealthy fats, and artificial ingredients. Instead, opt for whole, unprocessed foods that nourish your body and promote overall well-being.

6. Stay Hydrated: Drink plenty of water throughout the day. Water can help keep you hydrated, support digestion, and prevent overeating by curbing unnecessary snacking.

7. Regular Physical Activity: Incorporate regular exercise into your routine. Find activities you enjoy, such as walking, swimming, dancing, or yoga. Aim for at least 150 minutes of moderate-intensity exercise per week.

8. Stress Management: Chronic stress can contribute to weight gain and inflammation. Find healthy ways to manage stress, such as practicing mindfulness, deep breathing exercises, yoga, or engaging in hobbies you enjoy.

9. Seek Support: Surround yourself with a supportive network of friends, family, or even online communities that share similar goals. Having a support system can provide encouragement, accountability, and helpful tips along your weight loss journey.

10. Be Patient and Kind to Yourself: Remember that weight loss is a gradual process, and everyone's journey is unique. Focus on making sustainable lifestyle changes rather

than pursuing quick fixes. Be kind to yourself, celebrate small victories, and practice self-care along the way.

Approach your weight loss goals with a gentle and reassuring mindset. By adopting an anti-inflammatory diet and incorporating these lifestyle tips, you can create a sustainable and nourishing approach to losing weight while promoting overall health and well-being. Remember, it's about progress, not perfection. Listen to your body, honor your journey, and be proud of the positive changes you're making.

Nourishing Your Body - The Power of Anti-Inflammatory Nutrition

By understanding the nutrition-inflammation connection, we discover the power of anti-inflammatory foods, such as colorful fruits and vegetables, omega-3-rich fatty fish, wholesome grains, plant-based proteins, and inflammation-fighting spices. We also delve into the art of meal planning, providing tips for creating balanced, anti-inflammatory meals and meal prepping for success. Cooking with love and embracing culinary creativity is emphasized, encouraging readers to make anti-inflammatory meals exciting and delicious. The chapter also highlights the importance of involving loved ones, including children, in the cooking process to instill a love for wholesome foods from an early age. Through the exploration of nutrition and inflammation, we empower ourselves to support our bodies' healing processes and embark on a flavorful journey toward vibrant health.

Mastering the Kitchen - Essential Cooking Tools and Techniques

In this chapter, we embark on a culinary adventure, exploring the essential cooking tools and techniques that will empower us to create delicious, nourishing meals that support an anti-inflammatory lifestyle. With a fluid and human approach, we dive into the heart of the kitchen, equipping ourselves with the knowledge and skills needed to confidently prepare flavorful dishes.

We begin by discussing the must-have cooking tools that will make our culinary endeavors a breeze. From basic essentials like sharp knives, cutting boards, and measuring cups to more specialized tools such as high-quality cookware and food processors, we discover the key players that will enhance our cooking experience.

Through practical tips and guidance, we learn how to make the most of our kitchen tools and create a functional and efficient cooking space.

Next, we delve into fundamental cooking techniques that will elevate our culinary repertoire. We demystify techniques such as sautéing, roasting, steaming, and braising, providing step-by-step instructions that ensure success in the kitchen. With a reassuring tone, we encourage experimentation and emphasize that cooking should be a joyful and creative process. We learn to trust our instincts, taste as we go, and adapt recipes to suit our personal preferences.

To further enhance our cooking skills, we explore ingredient sourcing and emphasize the importance of quality ingredients in our anti-inflammatory journey. We discuss the benefits of organic and locally sourced produce, the value of selecting sustainable seafood, and the significance of choosing high-quality oils and spices. By understanding the origins of our ingredients and making thoughtful choices, we not only support our own health but also contribute to a more sustainable and ethical food system.

Throughout this chapter, we infuse our exploration of cooking tools and techniques with personal anecdotes and cultural insights. We celebrate the joy of shared meals and the memories that are created in the kitchen. Additionally, we provide nutritional information and highlight the health benefits of certain cooking methods and ingredient combinations, enriching the reader's experience with valuable knowledge.

By mastering essential cooking tools and techniques, we empower ourselves to create nourishing, flavorful meals that promote an anti-inflammatory lifestyle. With a fluid and human approach, we embrace the joy of cooking, infusing our dishes with love, creativity, and a deep understanding of the impact food can have on our well-being. Together, let's embark on this culinary journey and unleash our inner chef with confidence and reassurance.

Steaming:

Steaming is a gentle and health-conscious cooking method that preserves the natural flavors, colors, and nutrients of foods. It involves the use of steam to cook ingredients, without submerging them in water or oil. Steaming is perfect for delicate vegetables, seafood, and even grains like quinoa. By steaming our ingredients, we ensure that they retain their natural moisture and texture, resulting in vibrant and nutritious dishes. It's a simple yet effective technique that requires minimal effort and allows us to create light and flavorful meals.

Grilling:

Grilling is a popular cooking technique that adds a distinct smoky flavor to our food. It involves cooking ingredients directly over an open flame or on a hot grill pan. Grilling is not only a fantastic way to cook meats and poultry, but it also works wonders with vegetables and even fruits. The high heat of the grill creates a beautiful caramelization and enhances the natural flavors of the ingredients. Whether we're enjoying a juicy grilled steak or a charred vegetable skewer, grilling adds a delightful touch of outdoor cooking to our meals.

Braising:

Braising is a cooking technique that combines both dry and moist heat to create tender and flavorful dishes. It involves searing ingredients in a hot pan to develop a rich crust, and then slowly simmering them in a flavorful liquid, such as broth or wine. Braising is particularly suitable for tougher cuts of meat, such as beef or lamb, as the slow cooking process helps break down their fibers and infuse them with delicious flavors. The result is melt-in-your-mouth goodness that will leave your taste buds satisfied.

Sautéing:

Sautéing is a quick and versatile cooking technique that involves cooking ingredients over high heat in a small amount of fat, such as oil or butter. It's a fantastic way to bring out the flavors of vegetables, meats, and seafood in a short amount of time. By sautéing, we can achieve a perfect balance between caramelization and tenderness, resulting in dishes that are both flavorful and nutritious. From stir-fries to pan-seared fish fillets, sautéing allows us to create delicious meals with minimal fuss.

Baking:

Baking is a classic cooking technique that brings warmth and comfort to our kitchen. It involves cooking ingredients in an enclosed space, usually an oven, using dry heat. Baking is perfect for bread, pastries, casseroles, and even roasted vegetables. The controlled heat of the oven allows ingredients to cook evenly, develop beautiful textures, and release enticing aromas. Whether we're baking a batch of homemade cookies or roasting a tender chicken, this technique adds a delightful touch to our culinary creations.

Each of these cooking techniques offers unique flavors and textures, allowing us to explore a wide range of culinary possibilities. By mastering these techniques, we unlock the potential to create mouthwatering dishes that showcase the best flavors of our ingredients. So, let's embrace the art of steaming, grilling, braising, sautéing, and baking, and elevate our cooking skills to new heights.

The best method of cooking

The best way to cook for an anti-inflammatory diet is to prioritize whole, nutrient-dense ingredients and adopt cooking methods that preserve their beneficial properties. Here's a breakdown of the best cooking practices for an anti-inflammatory diet:

1. Choose Fresh, Whole Foods: Opt for fresh fruits, vegetables, lean proteins, and healthy fats. These whole foods are packed with essential nutrients and are less processed, minimizing potential inflammatory triggers.

2. Embrace Gentle Cooking Techniques: Use gentle cooking methods that retain the nutritional integrity of ingredients. Steaming, sautéing, and baking at moderate temperatures are ideal choices, as they help preserve the natural flavors, textures, and beneficial compounds in the food.

3. Limit High-Heat Cooking: Avoid deep-frying or cooking at extremely high temperatures, as it can lead to the formation of harmful compounds. Excessive heat can break down beneficial nutrients and generate pro-inflammatory substances. Instead, opt for lower heat methods that retain the food's nutritional value.

4. Incorporate Healthy Fats: Include anti-inflammatory fats such as olive oil, avocado oil, and coconut oil in your cooking. These fat are rich in antioxidants and can help reduce inflammation in the body. Avoid trans fats and minimize the use of vegetable oils high in omega-6 fatty acids, as they can promote inflammation.

5. Enhance Flavor Naturally: Use herbs, spices, and citrus juices to season your dishes instead of relying on excessive salt, sugar, or processed condiments. Herbs and spices like turmeric, ginger, garlic, and cinnamon have anti-inflammatory properties and can add depth and complexity to your meals.

6. Prioritize Plant-Based Foods: Aim to incorporate a variety of colorful fruits, vegetables, whole grains, legumes, and nuts into your recipes. Plant-based foods are rich in antioxidants, fiber, and phytonutrients, which can help reduce inflammation and support overall health.

7. Experiment with Anti-Inflammatory Ingredients: Include ingredients known for their anti-inflammatory properties, such as fatty fish rich in omega-3 fatty acids (salmon, mackerel), leafy greens, berries, walnuts, and flaxseeds. These ingredients can be incorporated into various recipes to enhance both flavor and health benefits.

8. Mindful Meal Preparation: Take time to plan and prepare your meals in advance. This helps you make conscious choices and avoid reaching for processed or unhealthy options when you're busy or tired. Batch cooking and meal prepping can be great strategies to ensure you have nutritious and inflammation-fighting meals readily available.

Remember, the key is to focus on wholesome, unprocessed foods, gentle cooking methods, and incorporating a variety of anti-inflammatory ingredients into your meals. By adopting these practices, you can support your overall health and well-being while enjoying delicious, nourishing meals.

Food and availability

Here's a list of ingredients for an anti-inflammatory diet, along with the best way to cook them, the best time to buy them in the USA, and whether they are quick or time-consuming to prepare. These ingredients can also be prepared with your children, making it a fun and educational experience:

Spinach:

- Best Cooking Method: Sauté or steam until wilted.

- Best Time to Buy: Year-round, but peak season is spring and fall.

- Cooking Time: Quick.

Blueberries:

- Best Cooking Method: Enjoy them fresh in smoothies, salads, or as a topping.

- Best Time to Buy: Summer.

- Cooking Time: No cooking required.

Salmon:

- Best Cooking Method: Grilling or baking for a flavorful and tender result.

- Best Time to Buy: Year-round.

- Cooking Time: Quick.

Turmeric:

- Best Cooking Method: Use as a spice in various dishes, such as curries or roasted vegetables.

- Best Time to Buy: Available year-round.

- Cooking Time: No cooking required.

Quinoa:

- Best Cooking Method: Rinse, then cook in boiling water or broth until tender.

- Best Time to Buy: Available year-round.

- Cooking Time: Moderate.

Ginger:

- Best Cooking Method: Grate or mince, then add to stir-fries, sauces, or teas.

- Best Time to Buy: Available year-round.

- Cooking Time: No cooking required.

Sweet Potatoes:

- Best Cooking Method: Roast or steam until tender.

- Best Time to Buy: Fall and winter.

- Cooking Time: Moderate.

Extra Virgin Olive Oil:

- Best Cooking Method: Use for salad dressings, drizzling over cooked vegetables, or sautéing at low to medium heat.

- Best Time to Buy: Available year-round.

- Cooking Time: No cooking required.

Walnuts:

- Best Cooking Method: Enjoy them as a snack, or chop and sprinkle on salads or oatmeal.

- Best Time to Buy: Available year-round.

- Cooking Time: No cooking required.

Dark Chocolate (70% cocoa or higher):

- Best Cooking Method: Enjoy as a treat or melt to make homemade chocolate-covered berries.

- Best Time to Buy: Available year-round.

- Cooking Time: No cooking required.

These ingredients provide a great foundation for an anti-inflammatory diet. They offer a wide range of flavors, textures, and health benefits. Cooking them with your children can be an enjoyable activity that helps teach them about nutritious food choices. Remember to involve them in age-appropriate tasks, such as washing produce, stirring ingredients, or measuring spices. Cooking together can create lasting memories and instill healthy habits from an early age.

By incorporating these ingredients into your meals, you can create delicious and nourishing dishes that support your overall well-being. Enjoy the process and savor the moments spent preparing and sharing these nutritious meals with your loved ones.

Forbidden foods

In an anti-inflammatory diet, it is recommended to limit or avoid certain foods that can promote inflammation in the body. While individual sensitivities may vary, here are some common foods to consider restricting or eliminating:

1. Processed and Refined Foods: These often contain high levels of 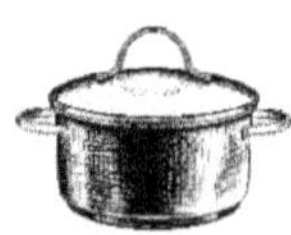 unhealthy fats, refined sugars, and artificial additives, which can contribute to inflammation. Examples include packaged snacks, sugary beverages, fast food, and processed meats.

2. Added Sugars: Excessive consumption of added sugars, such as those found in sugary drinks, desserts, and processed foods, can lead to increased inflammation and negatively impact overall health.

3. Trans Fats: Artificial trans fats, often found in fried and commercially baked goods, margarine, and some processed snacks, have been linked to inflammation and various health issues. It's best to avoid or minimize their intake.

4. High-Glycemic Index Foods: Foods that cause a rapid spike in blood sugar levels, such as refined grains (white bread, white rice) and sugary cereals, can contribute to inflammation. Opt for whole grains and low-glycemic index alternatives instead.

5. Vegetable Oils: Certain vegetable oils, such as soybean, corn, and sunflower oils, contain high levels of omega-6 fatty acids. While our bodies need a balance of omega-6 and omega-3 fatty acids, an excessive intake of omega-6s can promote inflammation. Use healthier alternatives like olive oil or avocado oil in moderation.

6. Artificial Additives: Food additives like artificial sweeteners, flavor enhancers (MSG), and preservatives may trigger inflammatory responses in some individuals. Choose whole, minimally processed foods whenever possible.

7. Excessive Alcohol: Heavy alcohol consumption can lead to inflammation and adversely affect overall health. Moderation is key if you choose to consume alcoholic beverages.

It's important to note that while these foods are generally associated with inflammation, individual tolerances may vary. Pay attention to how your body responds to certain foods and make adjustments based on your unique needs and sensitivities. A registered dietitian or healthcare professional can provide personalized guidance and support when following an anti-inflammatory diet.

A Guide to Navigating Restaurants on an Anti-Inflammatory Diet

Congratulations on your commitment to an anti-inflammatory diet! As you embark on this journey, you may encounter situations where dining out becomes a part of your social or professional life. While dining at a restaurant can present its challenges, fear not! With a little preparation and mindful choices, you can still enjoy delicious meals while sticking to your anti-inflammatory principles. Here's your guide to navigating restaurants with confidence:

1. Do Your Research: Before heading out, take the time to research the restaurant's menu online. Look for options that align with your anti-inflammatory goals. Many restaurants now offer online menus with detailed descriptions, making it easier to identify dishes that incorporate fresh, whole ingredients.

2. Choose the Right Restaurant: Opt for 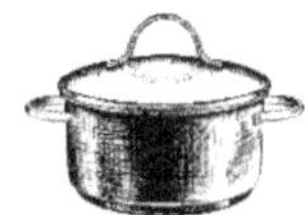 restaurants that emphasize healthy, organic, and locally sourced ingredients. Farm-to-table establishments or those with a focus on plant-based cuisine are often great options. These types of restaurants are more likely to have dishes that are prepared with minimal processing and inflammation-triggering ingredients.

3. Be Mindful of Portion Sizes: Restaurants often serve larger portions than what is necessary for a healthy meal. Consider sharing a dish with a dining companion or asking for a to-go box at the beginning of the meal to portion out what you don't plan to eat. This way, you can enjoy your meal without overindulging.

4. Communicate Your Dietary Needs: Don't be afraid to communicate your dietary preferences and restrictions to your server. Politely ask questions about ingredients, preparation methods, and customization options. Most restaurants are accommodating and can make adjustments to suit your needs. For example, you can ask for dressing or sauces on the side or substitute certain ingredients for healthier alternatives.

5. Prioritize Fresh, Whole Foods: Look for menu items that feature fresh vegetables, lean proteins, and whole grains. Opt for grilled, roasted, or steamed options instead of fried or breaded dishes. Choose salads with a variety of colorful vegetables, lean proteins like grilled chicken or fish, and dressings that are vinegar-based or oil and vinegar on the side.

6. Be Cautious with Sauces and Dressings: Many sauces and dressings in restaurants can be high in added sugars, unhealthy fats, and artificial ingredients. Ask for dressings on the side, so you can control the amount

you use. Alternatively, you can request simple options like olive oil, lemon juice, or balsamic vinegar to enhance the flavors of your meal.

7. Avoid Deep-Fried and Processed Foods: Deep-fried foods and processed menu items tend to be high in unhealthy fats, trans fats, and inflammatory additives. Steer clear of items like fried appetizers, breaded meats, and processed side dishes. Instead, opt for grilled, broiled, or baked options that are prepared with minimal added fats.

8. Watch out for Hidden Sugars: Many restaurant dishes, even savory ones, contain hidden sugars. Be mindful of menu items that are described as sweet, glazed, or smothered in sauces. Ask your server if there are added sugars in certain dishes and choose alternatives that are prepared with whole, natural ingredients.

9. Stay Hydrated: While dining out, it's important to stay hydrated. Opt for water or unsweetened herbal tea instead of sugary beverages. If you choose to enjoy an alcoholic beverage, do so in moderation and be aware that some cocktails can be high in added sugars and artificial ingredients.

10. Practice Mindful Eating: Slow down and savor each bite. Take the time to fully enjoy the flavors, textures, and aromas of your meal. Listen to your body's hunger and fullness cues and stop eating when you feel satisfied. Engage in mindful conversation with your dining companions, allowing yourself to fully experience the social aspect of dining out.

Remember, dining out should be an enjoyable experience. Embrace the opportunity to explore new flavors, support local restaurants, and savor the culinary delights while still adhering to your anti-inflammatory goals. By making mindful choices and advocating for your dietary needs, you can successfully navigate restaurants and continue your journey towards a healthier, more vibrant life.

Bon appétit and enjoy your dining adventures on the anti-inflammatory path!

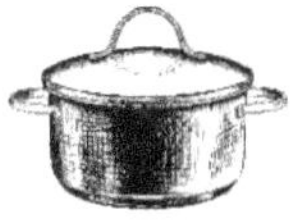

Breakfast

Turmeric Scrambled Eggs:

- Ingredients: 8 large eggs, 1 teaspoon ground turmeric, 1/2 teaspoon ground black pepper, 1 tablespoon olive oil, 2 tablespoons chopped fresh parsley.

- Directions: In a bowl, whisk together the eggs, turmeric, and black pepper. Heat olive oil in a skillet over medium heat. Pour in the egg mixture and cook, stirring gently, until the eggs are scrambled and cooked to your liking. Serve garnished with fresh parsley.

Chia Seed Pudding:

- Ingredients: 1/2 cup chia seeds, 2 cups almond milk, 1 tablespoon honey, 1 teaspoon vanilla extract, fresh berries for topping.

- Directions: In a bowl, mix together chia seeds, almond milk, honey, and vanilla extract. Stir well and let it sit in the refrigerator overnight or for at least 4 hours. Serve chilled with fresh berries on top.

Spinach and Mushroom Omelette:

- Ingredients: 8 large eggs, 1 cup baby spinach, 1 cup sliced mushrooms, 1/4 cup diced onion, 1 tablespoon olive oil, salt and pepper to taste.

- Directions: In a skillet, heat olive oil over medium heat. Add onions and mushrooms, and sauté until tender. Add spinach and cook until wilted. In a bowl, beat the eggs and season with salt and pepper. Pour the eggs over the vegetables in the skillet and cook until set. Fold the omelette in half and serve.

Green Smoothie Bowl:

- Ingredients: 2 frozen bananas, 1 cup fresh spinach, 1/2 cup almond milk, 1 tablespoon almond butter, 1 tablespoon honey, toppings of your choice (e.g., sliced fruits, nuts, seeds).

- Directions: In a blender, combine frozen bananas, spinach, almond milk, almond butter, and honey. Blend until smooth and creamy. Pour into a bowl and add your favorite toppings.

Avocado Toast with Smoked Salmon:

- Ingredients: 4 slices whole grain bread, 1 ripe avocado, smoked salmon slices, lemon juice, salt, and pepper to taste.

- Directions: Toast the bread slices. Mash the avocado in a bowl and add lemon juice, salt, and pepper. Spread the avocado mixture on the toasted bread and top with smoked salmon slices. Serve as an open-faced sandwich.

Quinoa Breakfast Bowl:

- Ingredients: 1 cup cooked quinoa, 1/2 cup almond milk, 1 tablespoon honey, 1/4 cup mixed berries, 1 tablespoon chopped nuts.

- Directions: In a bowl, combine cooked quinoa, almond milk, and honey. Stir well. Top with mixed berries and chopped nuts.

Sweet Potato and Kale Hash:

- Ingredients: 2 medium sweet potatoes (peeled and diced), 2 cups chopped kale, 1/2 onion (diced), 2 cloves garlic (minced), 1 tablespoon olive oil, salt, and pepper to taste.

- Directions: Heat olive oil in a skillet over medium heat. Add onions and garlic, and sauté until fragrant. Add sweet potatoes and cook until tender. Stir in the chopped kale and cook until wilted. Season with salt and pepper.

Berry Parfait:

- Ingredients: 2 cups Greek yogurt, 1 cup mixed berries, 1/4 cup granola, 1 tablespoon honey.

- Directions: In a glass or bowl, layer Greek yogurt, mixed berries, and granola. Drizzle with honey on top.

Buckwheat Pancakes:

- Ingredients: 1 cup buckwheat flour, 1/2 cup almond milk, 2 tablespoons honey, 1 teaspoon baking powder, 1/4 teaspoon salt, 2 eggs, 1 tablespoon coconut oil (melted).

- Directions: In a bowl, whisk together buckwheat flour, almond milk, honey, baking powder, salt, eggs, and melted coconut oil. Heat a non-stick skillet over medium heat and pour 1/4 cup of the batter onto the skillet. Cook until bubbles form on the surface, then flip and cook the other side until golden brown.

Breakfast Quinoa Bowl:

- Ingredients: 1 cup cooked quinoa, 1/2 cup almond milk, 1 tablespoon maple syrup, 1/4 cup sliced almonds, 1/4 cup dried cranberries, 1 teaspoon cinnamon.

- Directions: In a bowl, mix together cooked quinoa, almond milk, maple syrup, sliced almonds, dried cranberries, and cinnamon. Stir well and serve warm.

Ginger Turmeric Smoothie:

- Ingredients: 1 cup unsweetened almond milk, 1 ripe banana, 1-inch piece of fresh ginger (peeled and grated), 1 teaspoon ground turmeric, 1 tablespoon chia seeds, 1 tablespoon honey, ice cubes (optional).

- Directions: In a blender, combine almond milk, banana, grated ginger, turmeric, chia seeds, and honey. Blend until smooth. If desired, add ice cubes for a chilled texture. Pour into glasses and enjoy.

Kale and Tomato Frittata:

- Ingredients: 8 large eggs, 1 cup chopped kale, 1 cup cherry tomatoes (halved), 1/2 cup diced red bell pepper, 1/4 cup diced onion, 1 tablespoon olive oil, salt, and pepper to taste.

- Directions: Preheat the oven to 350°F (175°C). In a bowl, beat the eggs and season with salt and pepper. Heat olive oil in an oven-safe skillet over medium heat. Add onions and bell peppers, and sauté until softened. Stir in kale and cherry tomatoes. Pour the beaten eggs over the vegetables and gently stir to distribute evenly. Cook on the stovetop for a few minutes until the edges start to set. Transfer the skillet to the preheated oven and bake for about 10-12 minutes, or until the frittata is set. Slice into wedges and serve.

Almond Butter Overnight Oats:

- Ingredients: 1 cup rolled oats, 1 cup unsweetened almond milk, 2 tablespoons almond butter, 1 tablespoon honey, 1/4 cup sliced almonds, 1/4 cup fresh berries for topping.

- Directions: In a jar or container, combine rolled oats, almond milk, almond butter, and honey. Stir well to mix. Cover and refrigerate overnight. In the morning, give it a good stir and top with sliced almonds and fresh berries.

Smashed Avocado Toast with Poached Eggs:

- Ingredients: 4 slices whole grain bread, 2 ripe avocados, 4 poached eggs, 1 tablespoon lemon juice, salt, and pepper to taste, red pepper flakes for garnish (optional).

- Directions: Toast the bread slices. In a bowl, smash the avocados with lemon juice, salt, and pepper. Spread the avocado mixture onto the toasted bread. Top each slice with a poached egg. Sprinkle with red pepper flakes for a touch of heat.

Quinoa Breakfast Burrito:

- Ingredients: 1 cup cooked quinoa, 4 whole wheat tortillas, 4 large eggs (scrambled), 1/2 cup black beans (rinsed and drained), 1/4 cup diced red onion, 1/4 cup chopped fresh cilantro, salsa or hot sauce for serving.

- Directions: Warm the tortillas in a skillet or microwave. Fill each tortilla with scrambled eggs, cooked quinoa, black beans, diced red onion, and fresh cilantro. Roll up the tortillas to form burritos. Serve with salsa or hot sauce on the side.

Smoothie

Green Goddess Smoothie:

- Ingredients: :

  - 4 cups fresh spinach

  - 2 cups pineapple chunks

  - 2 ripe bananas

  - 1 tablespoon grated ginger

  - 1 tablespoon ground turmeric

  - 4 cups unsweetened almond milk

  - 1/4 cup walnuts

- Directions:

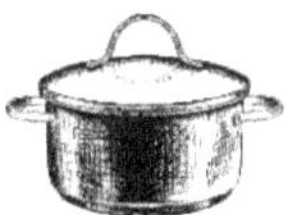

1. Place fresh spinach, pineapple chunks, ripe bananas, grated ginger, ground turmeric, and unsweetened almond milk in a blender.

2. Blend on high speed until smooth and creamy.

3. Add walnuts and blend again for a nutty texture.

- Description: This vibrant green smoothie is packed with anti-inflammatory powerhouses like spinach, pineapple, ginger, and turmeric. The addition of walnuts adds a delightful crunch and healthy fats to keep you satisfied.

- Calories: Approximately 250 per serving

- Tip: Use frozen pineapple chunks and pre-grated ginger for a quick and convenient preparation.

Berry Blast Smoothie:

- Ingredients:

  - 2 cups mixed berries (blueberries, strawberries, raspberries)

  - 2 cups fresh spinach

  - 2 ripe bananas

  - 4 cups unsweetened almond milk

  - 1 tablespoon cocoa powder

  - 1 tablespoon honey or maple syrup

- Directions:

  1. Combine mixed berries, fresh spinach, ripe bananas, unsweetened almond milk, cocoa powder, and honey or maple syrup in a blender.

  2. Blend until smooth and well combined.

- Description: This berry-packed smoothie is a delicious way to kick-start your day. The combination of mixed berries, spinach, cocoa powder, and almond milk provides a burst of antioxidants and a touch of sweetness.

- Calories: Approximately 200 per serving

- Tip: Freeze the ripe bananas in advance to create a creamy and chilled smoothie.

Citrus Sunshine Smoothie:

- Ingredients:

  - 4 oranges, peeled and segmented

  - 2 cups pineapple chunks

  - 2 cups fresh spinach

  - 4 cups green tea, chilled

  - Juice of 1 lemon

  - 1 tablespoon honey or maple syrup (optional)

- Directions:

1. Place orange segments, pineapple chunks, fresh spinach, chilled green tea, lemon juice, and honey or maple syrup (if desired) in a blender.

2. Blend until smooth and well combined.

- Description: This refreshing citrus smoothie is packed with vitamins and minerals from oranges, pineapple, spinach, and green tea. The zesty flavor and hydrating properties make it a perfect choice for a revitalizing drink.

- Calories: Approximately 150 per serving

- Tip: Use pre-cut oranges and frozen pineapple chunks for quick and easy preparation.

Tropical Turmeric Delight:

- Ingredients:

  - 2 cups fresh pineapple chunks

  - 1 ripe banana

  - 2 cups coconut water

  - 2 cups fresh spinach

  - 1 tablespoon grated ginger

  - 1 teaspoon ground turmeric

  - Juice of 1 lime

- Directions:

1. Combine fresh pineapple chunks, ripe banana, coconut water, fresh spinach, grated ginger, ground turmeric, and lime juice in a blender.

2. Blend until smooth and creamy.

- Description: This tropical-inspired smoothie combines the flavors of pineapple, banana, and coconut water with the anti-inflammatory properties of ginger and turmeric. It's a refreshing and vibrant blend that will transport you to a sunny paradise.

- Calories: Approximately 180 per serving

- Tip: Freeze the ripe banana in advance for a creamier texture and chill the coconut water for a refreshing twist.

Zesty Orange Ginger Smoothie:

- Ingredients:

  - 4 oranges, peeled and segmented

  - 1 large carrot, peeled and chopped

  - 1 tablespoon grated ginger

  - 2 cups fresh spinach

  - 2 cups almond milk

  - 1 tablespoon honey or maple syrup (optional)

- Directions:

  1. Place orange segments, chopped carrot, grated ginger, fresh spinach, almond milk, and honey or maple syrup (if desired) in a blender.

  2. Blend until smooth and well combined.

- Description: This zesty and energizing smoothie features the tangy flavor of oranges, the earthy sweetness of carrots, and the warming kick of ginger. Packed with antioxidants and vitamins, it's a delightful way to start your day.

- Calories: Approximately 140 per serving

- Tip: For a creamier texture, use almond milk that is unsweetened and fortified with calcium.

Scan the photo here

Enjoy these refreshing and nutrient-packed smoothies as part of your anti-inflammatory diet. They are not only delicious but also loaded with the goodness of anti-inflammatory ingredients. Cheers to your health and happy blending!

Green Power Smoothie:

- Ingredients:

  - 2 cups fresh spinach

  - 1 cup pineapple chunks

  - 1 ripe banana

- 1 tablespoon almond butter

- 1 cup almond milk

- Ice cubes (optional)

- Directions:

1. Add the fresh spinach, pineapple chunks, ripe banana, almond butter, and almond milk to a blender.

2. Blend on high speed until smooth and creamy.

3. If desired, add ice cubes and blend again for a chilled smoothie.

- Description: This vibrant green smoothie is packed with nutritious ingredients. The combination of spinach, pineapple, banana, almond butter, and almond milk provides a refreshing and energizing start to your day.

- Calories: Approximately 150 per serving

- Tip: Prepare and freeze individual smoothie packs in advance to streamline your morning routine. Simply blend the pre-portioned ingredients with almond milk when you're ready to enjoy.

Berry Beet Bliss Smoothie:

Scan the photo here

- Ingredients:

- 2 cups fresh or frozen mixed berries (blueberries, strawberries, raspberries)

- 1 small cooked beet, peeled and diced

- 1 cup plain Greek yogurt

- 1 tablespoon chia seeds

- 1 cup unsweetened almond milk

- Directions:

1. Place the mixed berries, cooked beet, Greek yogurt, chia seeds, and almond milk in a blender.

2. Blend until smooth and well combined.

- Description: This vibrant and antioxidant-rich smoothie combines the sweetness of mixed berries with the earthy flavors of beets. The addition of Greek yogurt and chia seeds adds a creamy texture and a boost of protein.

- Calories: Approximately 200 per serving

- Tip: If using fresh berries, add a handful of ice cubes to the blender for a chilled smoothie.

Tropical Paradise Smoothie:

Scan the photo here

- Ingredients:

  - 2 cups fresh or frozen pineapple chunks

  - 1 ripe banana

  - 1 cup coconut milk

  - 1 tablespoon fresh lime juice

  - 1 tablespoon shredded coconut (optional)

- Directions:

  1. Combine the pineapple chunks, ripe banana, coconut milk, and lime juice in a blender.

  2. Blend until smooth and creamy.

  3. Sprinkle with shredded coconut, if desired.

- Description: Transport yourself to a tropical paradise with this refreshing smoothie. The combination of sweet pineapple, creamy banana, coconut milk, and zesty lime juice will make you feel like you're on vacation.

- Calories: Approximately 180 per serving

- Tip: For an extra frosty smoothie, use frozen pineapple chunks and add a handful of ice cubes to the blender.

Citrus Burst Smoothie:

- Ingredients:

  - 2 oranges, peeled and segmented

  - 1 ripe mango, peeled and diced

  - 1 cup fresh spinach

  - 1 cup unsweetened almond milk

  - 1 tablespoon honey (optional)

- Directions:

  1. Place the orange segments, diced mango, fresh spinach, almond milk, and honey (if using) in a blender.

  2. Blend until smooth and well blended.

- Description: This refreshing smoothie bursts with the flavors of citrus and sweet mango. The addition of spinach adds a nutritious boost, making it a perfect choice for a revitalizing breakfast or snack.

- Calories: Approximately 160 per serving

- Tip: Use frozen mango chunks for a chilled and slushy texture without the need for ice cubes.

Chocolate Avocado Delight Smoothie:

- Ingredients:

  - 1 ripe avocado, peeled and pitted

  - 2 tablespoons unsweetened cocoa powder

  - 2 cups unsweetened almond milk

  - 2 tablespoons honey or maple syrup

  - Ice cubes (optional)

- Directions:

  1. In a blender, combine the ripe avocado, cocoa powder, almond milk, and sweetener of choice.

  2. Blend until smooth and creamy.

3. Add ice cubes, if desired, and blend again for a chilled smoothie.

- Description: Indulge your chocolate cravings with this creamy and nutritious smoothie. The combination of avocado, cocoa powder, and almond milk creates a luscious treat that satisfies your sweet tooth while providing essential nutrients.

- Calories: Approximately 220 per serving

Green Power Smoothie:

- Ingredients:

  - 4 cups spinach leaves

  - 2 cups pineapple chunks

  - 2 ripe bananas

  - 4 tablespoons almond butter

  - 4 cups almond milk

  - Ice cubes (optional)

- Directions:

  1. Place spinach leaves, pineapple chunks, ripe bananas, almond butter, and almond milk in a blender.

  2. Blend on high speed until smooth and creamy.

  3. Add ice cubes if desired, and blend again for a chilled smoothie.

- Description: This invigorating smoothie is packed with nutrients and antioxidants. The combination of spinach, pineapple, banana, almond butter, and almond milk provides a refreshing and energizing start to your day.

- Calories: Approximately 250 per serving

- Tip: To save time, pre-portion and freeze the ingredients in individual packs for quick and convenient smoothie preparation.

Berry Beet Blast Smoothie:

- Ingredients:

  - 2 cups mixed berries (blueberries, strawberries, raspberries)

  - 2 small cooked beets, peeled and diced

  - 2 cups Greek yogurt

  - 4 tablespoons chia seeds

  - 4 cups unsweetened almond milk

- Directions:

  1. Combine mixed berries, cooked beets, Greek yogurt, chia seeds, and almond milk in a blender.

  2. Blend until smooth and well combined.

- Description: This vibrant smoothie is bursting with antioxidant-rich berries and the earthy sweetness of beets. The addition of Greek yogurt and chia seeds provides a creamy texture and an extra dose of protein.

- Calories: Approximately 220 per serving

- Tip: Use frozen mixed berries for a refreshing and frosty smoothie.

Sunshine Citrus Smoothie:

- Ingredients:

  - 4 oranges, peeled and segmented

  - 2 ripe mangoes, peeled and diced

  - 4 cups unsweetened orange juice

  - Ice cubes (optional)

- Directions:

  1. Place orange segments, diced mangoes, and orange juice in a blender.

  2. Blend until smooth and well blended.

  3. Add ice cubes if desired, and blend again for a chilled smoothie.

- Description: This sunny and citrusy smoothie is a delightful way to start your day. The combination of oranges, mangoes, and orange juice provides a refreshing and vitamin-packed boost.

- Calories: Approximately 180 per serving

- Tip: For added convenience, use pre-cut oranges and frozen mango chunks.

Cocoa Crunch Delight Smoothie:

- Ingredients:

  - 4 ripe bananas

  - 4 tablespoons unsweetened cocoa powder

  - 4 cups unsweetened almond milk

  - 4 tablespoons almond butter

  - 1 cup crushed almonds

- Directions:

  1. In a blender, combine ripe bananas, cocoa powder, almond milk, and almond butter.

  2. Blend until smooth and creamy.

  3. Garnish with crushed almonds for a delightful crunch.

Scan the photo here

- Description: Indulge your chocolate cravings with this rich and satisfying smoothie. The combination of bananas, cocoa powder, almond milk, and almond butter creates a decadent treat that is both nutritious and delicious.

- Calories: Approximately 280 per serving

- Tip: Freeze ripe bananas in advance to add a creamy and icy texture to the smoothie.

Tropical Green Tea Paradise Smoothie:

- Ingredients:

  - 4 cups fresh or frozen pineapple chunks

  - 4 cups fresh spinach

  - 4 cups brewed green tea, chilled

- 4 tablespoons honey or maple syrup

- 1 cup ice cubes

- Directions:

1. Combine pineapple chunks, fresh spinach, chilled green tea, honey or maple syrup, and ice cubes in a blender.

2. Blend until smooth and well combined.

- Description: This refreshing and antioxidant-packed smoothie combines the tropical flavors of pineapple with the health benefits of green tea. The addition of spinach adds a nutritious boost, making it a perfect choice for a revitalizing drink.

- Calories: Approximately 150 per serving

- Tip: Use frozen pineapple chunks and pre-brewed green tea to save time and ensure a chilled smoothie.

Enjoy these refreshing and nutrient-packed smoothies as part of your anti-inflammatory diet. They are not only delicious but also loaded with the goodness of anti-inflammatory ingredients. Cheers to your health and a happy blending adventure!

- Tip: To enhance the chocolate flavor, add a pinch of sea salt or a dash of vanilla extract to the blender.

Enjoy these refreshing and nourishing smoothies as part of your anti-inflammatory diet. They're not only delicious but also packed with the goodness of anti-inflammatory ingredients. Cheers to good health and culinary delight!

Appetizers and Snacks

Ginger Turmeric Almond Energy Balls

Ingredients:

- 4 ounce almonds

- 2 tablespoons ground flaxseeds

- 2 tablespoons honey

- 1 tablespoon almond butter

- 1 teaspoon ground ginger

- 1 teaspoon ground turmeric

- 1/2 teaspoon vanilla extract

- Pinch of sea salt

- Unsweetened shredded coconut (for rolling)

- Directions:

1. In a food processor, blend the almonds until finely ground.

2. Add the flaxseeds, honey, almond butter, ginger, turmeric, vanilla extract, and sea salt. Process until well combined.

3. Shape the mixture into small balls, about 1 inch in diameter.

4. Roll the balls in shredded coconut to coat.

5. Place the energy balls in the refrigerator for at least 1 hour to firm up.

6. These ginger turmeric almond energy balls are a nutritious and convenient snack to fuel your day.

Preparation Time: 15 minutes

Chilling Time: 1 hour

Calories: Approximately 100 calories per energy ball

Low-Fat Cheesy Spinach Stuffed Mushrooms

Ingredients:

- 10 medium-sized button mushrooms

- 1 cup fresh spinach, finely chopped

- 1/4 cup low-fat cottage cheese

- 2 tablespoons grated Parmesan cheese

- 1 clove garlic, minced

- 1/2 teaspoon dried oregano

- Salt and pepper to taste

Scan the photo here

- Directions:

1. Preheat the oven to 375°F (190°C).

2. Remove the stems from the mushrooms and set aside.

3. In a bowl, combine the chopped spinach, cottage cheese, Parmesan cheese, minced garlic, dried oregano, salt, and pepper. Mix well.

4. Stuff each mushroom cap with the spinach and cheese mixture.

5. Place the stuffed mushrooms on a baking sheet and bake for 15-20 minutes, or until the mushrooms are tender and the filling is lightly browned.

6. Allow the mushrooms to cool slightly before serving.

7. These low-fat cheesy spinach stuffed mushrooms are a delightful and flavorful appetizer option.

Preparation Time: 15 minutes

Cooking Time: 15-20 minutes

Calories: Approximately 25 calories per stuffed mushroom

Ginger Turmeric Walnut Bliss Balls

Ingredients:

- 4 ounce walnuts

- 2 tablespoons unsweetened cocoa powder

- 2 tablespoons honey

- 1 tablespoon coconut oil

- 1 teaspoon ground ginger

- 1 teaspoon ground turmeric

- Pinch of sea salt

- Unsweetened shredded coconut (for rolling)

- Directions:

1. In a food processor, pulse the walnuts until finely chopped.

2. Add the cocoa powder, honey, coconut oil, ginger, turmeric, and sea salt. Process until well combined.

3. Shape the mixture into small balls, about 1 inch in diameter.

4. Roll the balls in shredded coconut to coat.

5. Place the bliss balls in the refrigerator for at least 1 hour to firm up.

6. These ginger turmeric walnut bliss balls are a satisfying and nutrient-packed snack.

Preparation Time: 15 minutes

Chilling Time: 1 hour

Calories: Approximately 120 calories per bliss ball

Smoked Salmon and Avocado Cucumber Bites

Ingredients:

- 1 English cucumber, sliced into rounds

- 4 ounces smoked salmon

- 1 avocado, sliced

- Fresh dill for garnish

- Lemon juice (optional)

- Salt and pepper to taste

- Directions:

1. Lay out the cucumber slices on a serving platter.

2. Top each cucumber slice with a small piece of smoked salmon.

3. Place a slice of avocado on top of the salmon.

4. Garnish with fresh dill and drizzle with a little lemon juice (if desired).

5. Season with salt and pepper to taste.

6. These smoked salmon and avocado cucumber bites are a refreshing and elegant appetizer choice.

Preparation Time: 10 minutes

Calories: Approximately 30 calories per bite

Tomato and Basil Bruschetta

Ingredients:

- 4 slices of whole grain baguette

- 2 large tomatoes, diced

- 1/4 cup of fresh basil leaves, chopped

- 1 clove of garlic, minced

- 1 tablespoon of extra virgin olive oil

- Salt and pepper, to taste

- Directions:

Scan the photo here

1. Preheat your oven to 375°F (190°C).

2. Place the baguette slices on a baking sheet and lightly toast them in the oven for about 5 minutes, or until they become crispy.

3. In a bowl, combine the diced tomatoes, chopped basil, minced garlic, extra virgin olive oil, salt, and pepper. Mix well to combine all the flavors.

4. Remove the toasted baguette slices from the oven and let them cool slightly.

5. Spoon the tomato and basil mixture onto each slice of baguette, distributing it evenly.

6. Serve immediately and enjoy!

Cooking Time: 5 minutes

Preparation Time: 10 minutes

Quantity: Makes 4 bruschetta slices

Calories: Approximately 80 calories per serving (2 bruschetta slices)

Tip:- For extra flavor, you can rub the toasted baguette slices with a garlic clove before adding the tomato and basil mixture.

- Choose ripe and juicy tomatoes for the best flavor in your bruschetta.

- If desired, you can drizzle a bit of balsamic glaze or reduction over the tomato and basil topping for added sweetness and depth of flavor.

- Feel free to customize your bruschetta by adding other ingredients such as mozzarella cheese, olives, or roasted red peppers.

Lunch

These recipes incorporate anti-inflammatory foods, are packed with flavor, and are designed to promote overall wellness. Let's get cooking!

Quinoa Salad with Roasted Vegetables:

- Ingredients:

  - 2 cups cooked quinoa

  - 1 cup cherry tomatoes, halved

  - 1 cup diced cucumber

  - 1 cup roasted bell peppers, sliced

  - 1/4 cup chopped fresh parsley

  - 1/4 cup crumbled feta cheese

  - 2 tablespoons extra virgin olive oil

  - 1 tablespoon lemon juice

  - Salt and pepper to taste

Scan the photo here

- Directions:

  1. In a large bowl, combine the cooked quinoa, cherry tomatoes, cucumber, roasted bell peppers, parsley, and feta cheese.

  2. Drizzle with olive oil and lemon juice. Season with salt and pepper. Toss gently to combine.

  3. Serve chilled or at room temperature.

- Description: This vibrant and refreshing quinoa salad is loaded with colorful vegetables and tossed in a zesty dressing. It's a perfect light lunch option.

- Cooking time: 15 minutes

- Calories: Approximately 250 calories per serving

- Practical tips: Cook the quinoa in advance and store it in the refrigerator for a quick assembly. Add grilled chicken or chickpeas for extra protein.

Grilled Salmon with Mango Salsa:

- Ingredients:

  - 4 salmon fillets (4-6 ounces each)

  - 1 ripe mango, diced

  - 1/4 cup diced red onion

  - 1/4 cup chopped fresh cilantro

  - 1 jalapeno, seeded and minced

  - 1 tablespoon lime juice

  - Salt and pepper to taste

- Directions:

  1. Preheat the grill to medium-high heat.

  2. Season the salmon fillets with salt and pepper. Grill for 4-6 minutes per side, or until cooked through.

  3. In a bowl, combine the diced mango, red onion, cilantro, jalapeno, lime juice, salt, and pepper. Mix well.

  4. Serve the grilled salmon topped with mango salsa.

- Description: This succulent grilled salmon is paired with a refreshing mango salsa, providing a delightful combination of flavors and textures.

- Cooking time: 12-15 minutes

- Calories: Approximately 300 calories per serving

- Practical tips: Use a grilling basket or foil to prevent the salmon from sticking to the grill. Serve with a side of steamed vegetables or quinoa for a complete meal.

Asian-Inspired Chicken Lettuce Wraps:

- Ingredients:

  - 1 lb boneless, skinless chicken breasts, diced

  - 2 tablespoons low-sodium soy sauce

  - 1 tablespoon hoisin sauce

  - 1 tablespoon rice vinegar

  - 1 tablespoon sesame oil

  - 2 cloves garlic, minced

  - 1 teaspoon grated fresh ginger

  - 8 large lettuce leaves

  - 1/4 cup shredded carrots

  - 1/4 cup chopped fresh cilantro

- Directions:

  1. In a bowl, combine the diced chicken, soy sauce, hoisin sauce, rice vinegar, sesame oil, garlic, and ginger. Marinate for 15 minutes.

  2. Heat a skillet over medium-high heat. Add the marinated chicken and cook for 6-8 minutes, or until cooked through.

  3. Place a spoonful of cooked chicken in each lettuce leaf. Top with shredded carrots and fresh cilantro.

  4. Roll up the lettuce leaves and secure with toothpicks, if desired.

- Description: These flavorful chicken lettuce wraps are inspired by Asian cuisine, featuring a delicious combination of marinated chicken, fresh vegetables, and aromatic herbs.

- Cooking time: 20 minutes

- Calories: Approximately 200 calories per serving

- Practical tips: Use pre-washed lettuce leaves for convenience. Serve with a side of brown rice or quinoa for added sustenance.

Mediterranean Chickpea Salad:

- Ingredients:

  - 2 cans chickpeas, drained and rinsed

  - 1 cup cherry tomatoes, halved

  - 1/2 cup diced cucumber

  - 1/4 cup chopped Kalamata olives

  - 1/4 cup crumbled feta cheese

  - 2 tablespoons chopped fresh parsley

  - 2 tablespoons lemon juice

  - 2 tablespoons extra virgin olive oil

  - Salt and pepper to taste

- Directions:

  1. In a large bowl, combine the chickpeas, cherry tomatoes, cucumber, Kalamata olives, feta cheese, and parsley.

  2. In a separate small bowl, whisk together the lemon juice, olive oil, salt, and pepper.

  3. Pour the dressing over the chickpea mixture and toss gently to coat.

  4. Serve chilled or at room temperature.

- Description: This refreshing Mediterranean chickpea salad showcases the flavors of the Mediterranean region, with a harmonious blend of ingredients and a zesty dressing.

- Cooking time: 10 minutes

- Calories: Approximately 250 calories per serving

- Practical tips: Use canned chickpeas for convenience. Add diced red onion or bell peppers for extra crunch.

Roasted Vegetable and Goat Cheese Frittata:

- Ingredients:

Scan the photo here

  - 8 large eggs

  - 1/4 cup milk

  - 1 cup diced roasted vegetables (such as bell peppers, zucchini, and eggplant)

  - 1/4 cup crumbled goat cheese

  - 2 tablespoons chopped fresh basil

  - Salt and pepper to taste

  - 1 tablespoon olive oil

- Directions:

  1. Preheat the oven to 375°F (190°C).

  2. In a bowl, whisk together the eggs, milk, salt, and pepper.

  3. Heat an ovenproof skillet over medium heat. Add the olive oil and roasted vegetables, sauté for 2-3 minutes.

  4. Pour the egg mixture over the vegetables. Sprinkle with crumbled goat cheese and chopped basil.

5. Transfer the skillet to the preheated oven and bake for 15-18 minutes, or until the frittata is set in the center.

6. Slice and serve warm or at room temperature.

- Description: This savory frittata is packed with roasted vegetables and creamy goat cheese, offering a delightful combination of flavors and textures.

- Cooking time: 25 minutes

- Calories: Approximately 200 calories per serving

- Practical tips: Use leftover roasted vegetables to save time. Customize the frittata by adding your favorite herbs or spices.

Sweet Potato and Black Bean Tacos:

- Ingredients:

  - 4 small sweet potatoes, peeled and diced

  - 1 can black beans, drained and rinsed

  - 1 teaspoon chili powder

  - 1/2 teaspoon cumin

  - 1/2 teaspoon paprika

  - Salt and pepper to taste

  - 8 small corn tortillas

  - Toppings: diced avocado, chopped cilantro, lime wedges

- Directions:

1. Preheat the oven to 400°F (200°C). Place the diced sweet potatoes on a baking sheet and drizzle with olive oil. Sprinkle with chili powder, cumin, paprika, salt, and pepper. Toss to coat evenly. Roast for 20-25 minutes, or until the sweet potatoes are tender.

2. In a small saucepan, heat the black beans over medium heat. Season with salt and pepper, and stir in a pinch of chili powder for added flavor.

3. Warm the corn tortillas in a dry skillet or microwave.

4. To assemble the tacos, spoon a portion of roasted sweet potatoes and black beans onto each tortilla. Top with diced avocado and chopped cilantro. Squeeze fresh lime juice over the filling.

5. Serve the tacos warm.

- Description: These vegetarian sweet potato and black bean tacos are bursting with flavor and textures. The roasted sweet potatoes and seasoned black beans create a satisfying and nutritious filling.

- Cooking time: 30 minutes

- Calories: Approximately 250 calories per serving

- Practical tips: Pre-cook the sweet potatoes and black beans in advance for quicker assembly. Add a dollop of Greek yogurt or a sprinkle of cheese for extra creaminess.

Ginger-Turmeric Chicken Stir-Fry:

- Ingredients:

  - 1 lb boneless, skinless chicken breasts, thinly sliced

  - 1 tablespoon grated fresh ginger

  - 1 tablespoon grated fresh turmeric (or 1 teaspoon ground turmeric)

  - 2 cloves garlic, minced

  - 2 tablespoons low-sodium soy sauce

  - 1 tablespoon honey or maple syrup

  - 2 tablespoons sesame oil

  - 1 tablespoon olive oil

Scan the photo here

- 2 cups mixed vegetables (such as bell peppers, broccoli, and snap peas)

- Sesame seeds for garnish

- Directions:

1. In a bowl, combine the sliced chicken, grated ginger, grated turmeric, minced garlic, soy sauce, and honey. Let it marinate for 15 minutes.

2. Heat the olive oil and sesame oil in a large skillet or wok over medium-high heat. Add the marinated chicken and stir-fry for 5-7 minutes, or until cooked through.

3. Add the mixed vegetables to the skillet and stir-fry for an additional 3-4 minutes, or until crisp-tender.

4. Sprinkle with sesame seeds for garnish.

5. Serve the ginger-turmeric chicken stir-fry over brown rice or quinoa.

- Description: This vibrant stir-fry combines the aromatic flavors of ginger and turmeric with tender chicken and a colorful assortment of vegetables. It's a delicious and nutritious lunch option.

- Cooking time: 20 minutes

- Calories: Approximately 300 calories per serving

- Practical tips: Use pre-grated ginger and turmeric for convenience. Adjust the sweetness by adding more or less honey/maple syrup.

Kale and White Bean Soup:

- Ingredients:

  - 2 tablespoons olive oil

  - 1 onion, diced

  - 3 cloves garlic, minced

- 4 cups vegetable broth

- 1 can diced tomatoes

- 2 cups chopped kale

- 1 can white beans, drained and rinsed

- 1 teaspoon dried oregano

- 1/2 teaspoon dried thyme

- Salt and pepper to taste

- Directions:

1. In a large pot, heat the olive oil over medium heat. Add the diced onion and minced garlic. Sauté until the onion becomes translucent.

2. Pour in the vegetable broth and diced tomatoes. Bring to a boil.

3. Add the chopped kale, white beans, dried oregano, dried thyme, salt, and pepper. Simmer for 15-20 minutes, or until the kale is tender.

4. Adjust the seasoning if needed.

5. Serve the kale and white bean soup hot with a sprinkle of freshly grated Parmesan cheese, if desired.

- Description: This hearty and comforting kale and white bean soup is packed with nutritious ingredients and warming flavors. It's a satisfying lunch choice, especially on cooler days.

- Cooking time: 30 minutes

- Calories: Approximately 250 calories per serving

- Practical tips: Use pre-washed and pre-chopped kale to save time. Add a squeeze of lemon juice before serving for a refreshing touch.

Salmon and Avocado Salad:

- Ingredients:

   - 4 salmon fillets (4-6 ounces each)

   - 4 cups mixed salad greens

   - 1 avocado, sliced

   - 1/2 cup cherry tomatoes, halved

   - 1/4 cup sliced red onion

   - 2 tablespoons lemon juice

   - 2 tablespoons extra virgin olive oil

   - Salt and pepper to taste

- Directions:

   1. Preheat the oven to 400°F (200°C). Place the salmon fillets on a baking sheet lined with parchment paper. Season with salt and pepper. Bake for 12-15 minutes, or until cooked through.

   2. In a large bowl, combine the mixed salad greens, avocado slices, cherry tomatoes, and sliced red onion.

   3. In a separate small bowl, whisk together the lemon juice, olive oil, salt, and pepper.

   4. Drizzle the dressing over the salad mixture and toss gently to coat.

   5. Divide the salad onto plates and top each portion with a baked salmon fillet.

- Description: This delightful salmon and avocado salad offers a perfect balance of flavors and textures. It's a light and refreshing lunch option.

- Cooking time: 15 minutes

- Calories: Approximately 300 calories per serving

- Practical tips: Use canned salmon for a quicker assembly. Add a sprinkle of toasted nuts or seeds for extra crunch.

Spinach and Walnut Salad:

- Ingredients:

  - 8 cups baby spinach leaves

  - 1 cup chopped walnuts

  - 1 cup cherry tomatoes, halved

  - 1/4 cup crumbled feta cheese

  - 2 tablespoons extra virgin olive oil

  - 2 tablespoons balsamic vinegar

  - Salt and pepper to taste

- Directions:

  1. In a large salad bowl, combine the baby spinach leaves, chopped walnuts, cherry tomatoes, and crumbled feta cheese.

  2. Drizzle the extra virgin olive oil and balsamic vinegar over the salad.

  3. Season with salt and pepper, then toss everything together until well combined.

- Description: This refreshing and nutrient-packed salad features vibrant baby spinach leaves, crunchy walnuts, juicy cherry tomatoes, and creamy feta cheese. The combination of flavors and textures makes it a delightful lunch option.

- Preparation time: 10 minutes

- Calories: Approximately 250 per serving

- Tip: To save time, you can wash and dry the spinach leaves in advance or use pre-washed baby spinach from the grocery store.

Salmon and Avocado Wrap:

- Ingredients:

  - 4 whole wheat tortilla wraps

- 4 salmon fillets (4 ounces each), cooked and flaked

- 2 ripe avocados, sliced

- 1 cup baby spinach leaves

- 1/4 cup Greek yogurt

- Juice of 1 lemon

- Salt and pepper to taste

- Directions:

1. Lay out the whole wheat tortilla wraps on a clean surface.

2. Spread Greek yogurt on each wrap, leaving a border around the edges.

3. Top with cooked and flaked salmon, avocado slices, and baby spinach leaves.

4. Squeeze lemon juice over the fillings and season with salt and pepper.

5. Roll up the wraps tightly, tucking in the sides as you go.

6. Cut each wrap in half diagonally before serving.

- Description: This flavorful and nourishing wrap combines the richness of flaked salmon, the creaminess of avocado slices, and the freshness of baby spinach. It's a satisfying and portable lunch option.

- Preparation time: 15 minutes

- Calories: Approximately 350 per serving

- Tip: To speed up the preparation, you can use leftover cooked salmon or opt for canned salmon instead.

Broccoli and Quinoa Salad

- Ingredients:

- 2 cups cooked quinoa

- 2 cups steamed broccoli florets

- 1/2 cup diced tomatoes

- 1/4 cup diced red onion

- 1/4 cup chopped fresh parsley

- 2 tablespoons lemon juice

- 2 tablespoons extra virgin olive oil

- Salt and pepper to taste

- Directions:

1. In a large mixing bowl, combine the cooked quinoa, steamed broccoli florets, diced tomatoes, diced red onion, and chopped parsley.

2. Drizzle the lemon juice and extra virgin olive oil over the salad.

3. Season with salt and pepper, then toss everything together until well coated.

- Description: This vibrant salad brings together the nutty flavors of quinoa, the crispness of steamed broccoli, and the tanginess of tomatoes. It's a satisfying and nutritious lunch option that's packed with anti-inflammatory ingredients.

- Preparation time: 20 minutes

- Calories: Approximately 200 per serving

- Tip: Cook a batch of quinoa and steam the broccoli in advance to have them ready for quick assembly.

Beetroot and Orange Salad:

- Ingredients:

- 4 medium beets, cooked and sliced

- 2 oranges, peeled and segmented

- 1/4 cup chopped walnuts

- 1/4 cup crumbled goat cheese

- 2 tablespoons balsamic vinegar

- 1 tablespoon honey

- 1 tablespoon extra -virgin olive oil

- Directions:

1. In a large salad bowl, combine the cooked and sliced beets, orange segments, chopped walnuts, and crumbled goat cheese.

2. In a small bowl, whisk together the balsamic vinegar, honey, and extra virgin olive oil to make the dressing.

3. Drizzle the dressing over the salad ingredients and toss gently to coat.

- Description: This colorful salad features the earthy sweetness of beets, the refreshing citrus flavors of oranges, the crunch of walnuts, and the tanginess of goat cheese. It's a vibrant and nutrient-dense lunch option.

- Preparation time: 15 minutes

- Calories: Approximately 300 per serving

- Tip: Use pre-cooked and sliced beets available in the grocery store to save time on cooking and preparation.

Tuna and Blueberry Salad:

- Ingredients:

  - 4 cups mixed salad greens

  - 2 cans tuna in water, drained

  - 1 cup fresh blueberries

  - 1/4 cup sliced almonds

  - 2 tablespoons lemon juice

  - 1 tablespoon extra- virgin olive oil

  - Salt and pepper to taste

- Directions:

1. In a large salad bowl, combine the mixed salad greens, drained tuna, fresh blueberries, and sliced almonds.

2. In a small bowl, whisk together the lemon juice, extra virgin olive oil, salt, and pepper to make the dressing.

3. Drizzle the dressing over the salad ingredients and toss gently to coat.

- Description: This refreshing salad pairs protein-rich tuna with antioxidant-packed blueberries, creating a delightful combination of flavors. The addition of mixed salad greens and sliced almonds adds crunch and texture.

- Preparation time: 10 minutes

- Calories: Approximately 250 per serving

- Tip: Opt for wild-caught tuna packed in water for a healthier choice, and use pre-washed salad greens for convenience.

These lunch recipes provide a delicious way to incorporate anti-inflammatory foods into your diet. Enjoy these flavorful and nutritious meals that will support your well-being while keeping your taste buds satisfied.

Turkey and Vegetable Lettuce Wraps:

- Ingredients:

  - 1 lb ground turkey

  - 1 tablespoon olive oil

  - 1/2 cup diced bell peppers

  - 1/2 cup diced zucchini

  - 1/2 cup diced carrots

  - 2 cloves garlic, minced

  - 1 teaspoon grated fresh ginger

  - 2 tablespoons low-sodium soy sauce

  - 1 tablespoon hoisin sauce

  - 1 tablespoon rice vinegar

  - 8 large lettuce leaves

  - Optional toppings: sliced green onions, chopped peanuts

Scan the photo here

- Directions:

  1. Heat the olive oil in a large skillet over medium heat. Add the ground turkey and cook until browned.

  2. Add the diced bell peppers, zucchini, carrots, minced garlic, and grated ginger to the skillet. Sauté for 5-7 minutes, or until the vegetables are tender.

3. In a small bowl, whisk together the soy sauce, hoisin sauce, and rice vinegar. Pour the sauce over the turkey and vegetable mixture. Stir to combine and cook for an additional 2-3 minutes.

4. Spoon the turkey and vegetable mixture onto lettuce leaves. Top with sliced green onions and chopped peanuts, if desired.

5. Roll up the lettuce leaves and enjoy.

- Description: These turkey and vegetable lettuce wraps are a delicious and nutritious option for a satisfying lunch. Combining ground turkey and colorful vegetables creates a flavorful filling, while the crisp lettuce leaves provide a refreshing crunch.

- Cooking time: 20 minutes

- Calories: Approximately 250 calories per serving

- Practical tips: To save time, you can prep the vegetables in advance and store them in the refrigerator. If you prefer a spicier flavor, add a dash of hot sauce or chili flakes to the turkey mixture. Get your family involved by letting them assemble their own lettuce wraps and customize the toppings.

Pasta

Spinach and Walnut Pasta:

- Ingredients:

  - 12ounce whole wheat pasta

  - 2 cups fresh spinach

  - 1 cup walnuts, chopped

  - 1 cup cherry tomatoes, halved

  - 2 cloves garlic, minced

  - 2 tablespoons extra virgin olive oil

  - Salt and pepper to taste

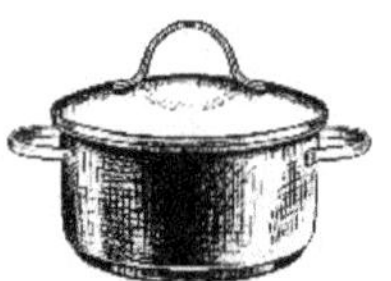

- Directions:

  1. Cook the pasta according to package instructions until al dente. Drain and set aside.

  2. In a large pan, heat the olive oil over medium heat. Add minced garlic and sauté until fragrant.

  3. Add spinach and cook until wilted. Stir in cherry tomatoes and walnuts.

  4. Add the cooked pasta to the pan and toss until well combined. Season with salt and pepper.

- Description: This pasta dish combines the nuttiness of walnuts with the vibrant flavors of spinach and cherry tomatoes. It's a wholesome and satisfying meal that's rich in anti-inflammatory ingredients.

- Cooking Time: Approximately 20 minutes

- Calories: Approximately 400 per serving

- Tip: Toast the walnuts in a dry skillet for a few minutes to enhance their flavor before adding them to the dish.

Roasted Vegetable Pasta:

- Ingredients:

  - 12ounce whole wheat pasta

  - 2 cups broccoli florets

  - 1 cup diced fresh beets

  - 1 cup cherry tomatoes, halved

  - 2 tablespoons extra virgin olive oil

  - 2 cloves garlic, minced

  - Salt and pepper to taste

- Directions:

  1. Preheat the oven to 400°F (200°C). Toss the broccoli florets, diced beets, and cherry tomatoes with olive oil, minced garlic, salt, and pepper. Spread them on a baking sheet and roast for about 20 minutes, or until tender.

  2. Cook the pasta according to package instructions until al dente. Drain and set aside.

  3. In a large pan, combine the roasted vegetables and cooked pasta. Toss until well mixed.

- Description: This pasta dish showcases the deliciousness of roasted vegetables, including broccoli, beets, and cherry tomatoes. It's a colorful and nutrient-rich meal that will satisfy your taste buds and nourish your body.

- Cooking Time: Approximately 30 minutes

- Calories: Approximately 380 per serving

- Tip: Add a sprinkle of grated Parmesan cheese or a drizzle of balsamic glaze for an extra burst of flavor.

Salmon and Tomato Pasta:

- Ingredients:

  - 12ounce whole wheat pasta

  - 4 salmon fillets (6 ounces each), cooked and flaked

  - 2 cups cherry tomatoes, halved

  - 2 tablespoons extra virgin olive oil

  - 2 cloves garlic, minced

  - 1 teaspoon dried basil

  - Salt and pepper to taste

- Directions:

  1. Cook the pasta according to package instructions until al dente. Drain and set aside.

  2. In a large pan, heat the olive oil over medium heat. Add minced garlic and sauté until fragrant.

  3. Add cherry tomatoes to the pan and cook until they start to soften. Stir in the cooked and flaked salmon.

  4. Add the cooked pasta to the pan and toss until well coated. Season with dried basil, salt, and pepper.

- Description: This pasta dish combines the heart-healthy benefits of salmon with the burst of flavor from cherry tomatoes. It's a satisfying and nutritious meal that will leave you feeling satisfied and nourished.

- Cooking Time: Approximately 20 minutes

- Calories: Approximately 420 per serving

- Tip: Sprinkle some freshly chopped basil or parsley on top before serving for a vibrant and fresh taste.

Turmeric Ginger Carrot Pasta:

- Ingredients:

  - 12ounce whole wheat pasta

  - 2 cups grated carrots

  - 2 cloves garlic, minced

  - 1 tablespoon grated ginger

  - 2 tablespoons extra virgin olive oil

  - 1 teaspoon ground turmeric

  - Salt and pepper to taste

- Directions:

  1. Cook the pasta according to package instructions until al dente. Drain and set aside.

  2. In a large pan, heat the olive oil over medium heat. Add minced garlic and grated ginger. Sauté until fragrant.

  3. Add grated carrots to the pan and cook until tender. Stir in ground turmeric and season with salt and pepper.

  4. Add the cooked pasta to the pan and toss until well combined. Adjust the seasoning if needed.

- Description: This vibrant pasta dish features the anti-inflammatory power of turmeric and ginger, combined with the natural sweetness of carrots. It's a simple yet flavorful meal that will brighten up your day.

- Cooking Time: Approximately 25 minutes

- Calories: Approximately 360 per serving

- Tip: Add a squeeze of lemon juice or sprinkle some crushed red pepper flakes for a tangy or spicy kick.

Citrus Salmon Pasta Salad:

- Ingredients:

  - 12ounce whole wheat pasta, cooked and cooled

  - 4 salmon fillets (6 ounces each), cooked and flaked

  - 2 cups baby spinach

  - 1 cup cherry tomatoes, halved

  - Juice of 1 lemon

  - 2 tablespoons extra virgin olive oil

- Salt and pepper to taste

- Directions:

1. In a large bowl, combine the cooked and cooled pasta, flaked salmon, baby spinach, and cherry tomatoes.

2. In a small bowl, whisk together lemon juice, extra virgin olive oil, salt, and pepper to make a dressing.

3. Pour the dressing over the pasta mixture and toss until well coated. Adjust the seasoning if needed.

- Description: This refreshing pasta salad combines the goodness of salmon, baby spinach, and cherry tomatoes with the zesty flavors of citrus. It's a light and satisfying dish that's perfect for a quick and healthy lunch or dinner.

- Cooking Time: Approximately 15 minutes (plus cooling time for the pasta)

- Calories: Approximately 390 per serving

- Tip: Add some sliced almonds or toasted pine nuts for an extra crunch and a dose of healthy fats.

Enjoy these delightful and nutritious pasta recipes as part of your anti-inflammatory diet. They are designed to be both flavorful and packed with anti-inflammatory ingredients to support your well-being. Bon appétit!

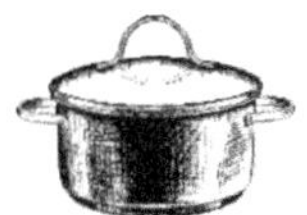

Snacks

Fresh Berry Parfait

Ingredients:

- 2 cups mixed berries (strawberries, blueberries, raspberries)

- 1 cup Greek yogurt

- 1 tablespoon honey

- ¼ cup granola

Description: In a bowl, layer the mixed berries with Greek yogurt. Drizzle honey on top and sprinkle granola for added crunch. This quick and easy parfait is packed with antioxidants from the berries and the probiotic benefits of Greek yogurt.

Calories: Approximately 150 calories per serving.

Practical tip: Prepare the parfait in advance and keep it refrigerated until ready to serve. It's a refreshing snack that can be enjoyed anytime.

Avocado Toast

Ingredients:

- 2 slices whole grain bread

- 1 ripe avocado
Scan the photo here

- Juice of 1 lemon

- Pinch of sea salt

- Optional toppings: sliced tomatoes, red pepper flakes

Description: Toast the bread until golden brown. Mash the avocado in a bowl and mix in lemon juice and sea salt. Spread the avocado mixture onto the toast. Top with sliced tomatoes and a sprinkle of red pepper flakes for added flavor.

Calories: Approximately 200 calories per serving.

Practical tip: To speed up the preparation, use pre-sliced bread and store-bought guacamole if you're short on time.

Cucumber Hummus Bites

Ingredients:

- 1 cucumber

- ½ cup hummus

- Fresh dill or parsley for garnish

Description: Slice the cucumber into thin rounds. Place a dollop of hummus on each cucumber slice. Garnish with fresh dill or parsley for added freshness.

Calories: Approximately 60 calories per serving.

Practical tip: Use a small melon baller to scoop out the center of each cucumber slice for a perfect bite-sized snack.

Greek Yogurt Dip with Veggies

Ingredients:

- 1 cup Greek yogurt

- 1 tablespoon lemon juice

- 1 teaspoon dried dill

- Assorted fresh vegetables (carrots, bell peppers, cucumber, celery) for dipping

Description: In a bowl, mix Greek yogurt, lemon juice, and dried dill until well combined. Serve the yogurt dip with an assortment of fresh vegetables for a crunchy and satisfying snack.

Calories: Approximately 100 calories per serving.

Practical tip: Prepare the dip in advance and keep it refrigerated. It can be enjoyed throughout the week with different vegetables.

Apple Slices with Almond Butter

Ingredients:

- 2 apples, sliced

- ¼ cup almond butter

- Optional toppings: cinnamon, chopped nuts

Description: Dip apple slices into almond butter for a delicious and nutritious snack. Sprinkle cinnamon or chopped nuts on top for extra flavor and texture.

Calories: Approximately 180 calories per serving.

Practical tip: Use pre-sliced apples if you're short on time. Keep the almond butter handy for a quick and easy snack option.

Chia Pudding

Ingredients:

- ¼ cup chia seeds

- 1 cup unsweetened almond milk

- 1 tablespoon honey or maple syrup

- Fresh berries for topping

Description: In a bowl, mix chia seeds, almond milk, and sweetener of your choice. Let it sit in the refrigerator for at least 2 hours or overnight. Serve with fresh berries on top.

Calories: Approximately 150 calories per serving.

Practical tip: Prepare the chia pudding the night before for a ready-to-eat snack in the morning.

Trail Mix

Ingredients:

- 1 cup mixed nuts (almonds, walnuts, cashews)

- ¼ cup dried fruit (raisins, cranberries, apricots)

- ¼ cup dark chocolate chips

- Optional: coconut flakes, pumpkin seeds

Description: Combine all ingredients in a bowl and mix well. Portion out into individual snack bags for a convenient on-the-go snack.

Calories: Approximately 200 calories per serving.

Practical tip: Make a large batch of trail mix and store it in an airtight container for quick and easy snacking throughout the week.

Greek Yogurt Berry Popsicles

Ingredients:

- 1 cup Greek yogurt

- ½ cup mixed berries (strawberries, blueberries, raspberries)

- 1 tablespoon honey or maple syrup

Description: In a blender, combine Greek yogurt, mixed berries, and sweetener. Blend until smooth. Pour the mixture into popsicle molds and freeze for at least 4 hours or until set.

Calories: Approximately 80 calories per serving.

Practical tip: Make a batch of popsicles in advance and have them ready for a refreshing and healthy snack option.

Rice Cake with Smashed Avocado

Ingredients:

- 4 rice cakes

- 1 ripe avocado

- Juice of 1 lime

- Pinch of sea salt

- Optional toppings: sliced cherry tomatoes, sprouts

Description: Lightly toast the rice cakes until crisp. Mash the avocado in a bowl and mix in lime juice and sea salt. Spread the avocado mixture onto the rice cakes. Top with sliced cherry tomatoes and sprouts for added freshness.

Calories: Approximately 120 calories per serving.

Practical tip: Keep a pack of rice cakes on hand for a quick and easy snack. Customize the toppings based on your preferences.

Vegetable Crudité with Yogurt Dip

Ingredients:

- Assorted fresh vegetables (carrots, bell peppers, cucumber, celery)

- 1 cup Greek yogurt

- 1 tablespoon lemon juice

- 1 teaspoon dried herbs (such as dill, parsley, or chives)

- Pinch of sea salt

Description: Slice the vegetables into sticks or bite-sized pieces. In a bowl, mix Greek yogurt, lemon juice, dried herbs, and sea salt. Serve the yogurt dip with the fresh vegetable crudité.

Calories: Approximately 80 calories per serving.

Practical tip: Prepare the vegetable sticks in advance and store them in a container with water to keep them fresh and crisp. The yogurt dip can be made ahead and refrigerated for convenience.

Pineapple and Blueberry Smoothie

Ingredients:

- 1 cup of pineapple chunks

- 1 cup of blueberries

- 1 cup of spinach leaves

- 1 cup of almond milk

- 1 tablespoon of chia seeds

- Ice cubes (optional)

Directions:

1. Place all the ingredients in a blender.

2. Blend until smooth and creamy.

3. If desired, add ice cubes and blend again until chilled.

4. Pour the smoothie into glasses and enjoy it as a refreshing and nutritious dinner option or a snack.

Calories: Approximately 150 per serving

Dinner

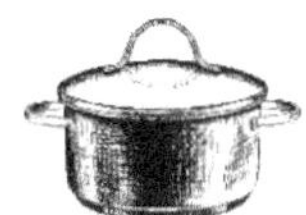

Baked Salmon with Roasted Vegetables:

- Ingredients: 4 salmon fillets (6 ounces each), 2 cups broccoli florets, 1 cup cherry tomatoes, 1 tablespoon olive oil, salt, and pepper to taste, lemon wedges for serving.

- Directions: Preheat the oven to 400°F (200°C). Place the salmon fillets on a baking sheet. Toss the broccoli florets and cherry tomatoes with olive oil, salt, and pepper, then spread them around the salmon on the baking sheet. Bake for about 15-20 minutes, or until the salmon is cooked through and the vegetables are tender. Serve with lemon wedges.

Spinach and Quinoa Stuffed Bell Peppers:

- Ingredients: 4 bell peppers, 1 cup cooked quinoa, 2 cups fresh spinach leaves, 1/2 cup diced tomatoes, 1/4 cup diced red onion, 1/4 cup crumbled feta cheese, 1 tablespoon olive oil, salt, and pepper to taste.

- Directions: Preheat the oven to 375°F (190°C). Cut the tops off the bell peppers and remove the seeds and membranes. In a bowl, combine cooked quinoa, spinach, diced tomatoes, red onion, feta cheese, olive oil, salt, and pepper. Stuff the bell peppers with the quinoa mixture. Place the stuffed peppers in a baking dish and bake for about 25-30 minutes, or until the peppers are tender and the filling is heated through.

Tomato Basil Chicken Skewers:

- Ingredients: 4 boneless, skinless chicken breasts (cut into chunks), 1 cup cherry tomatoes, 1/4 cup fresh basil leaves, 2 tablespoons olive oil, 2 cloves garlic (minced), salt, and pepper to taste.

- Directions: Preheat the grill or grill pan over medium-high heat. Thread the chicken chunks, cherry tomatoes, and basil leaves onto skewers. In a small bowl, mix together olive oil, minced garlic, salt, and pepper. Brush the mixture onto the skewers. Grill the skewers for about 8-10 minutes, turning occasionally, until the chicken is cooked through. Serve hot.

Cocoa-Spiced Beef Stir-Fry:

- Ingredients: 1pound beef sirloin (sliced into thin strips), 2 cups broccoli florets, 1 red bell pepper (sliced), 1/2 cup sliced carrots, 2 tablespoons low-sodium soy sauce, 1 tablespoon cocoa powder, 1 teaspoon ground cumin, 1/2 teaspoon chili powder, 1/2 teaspoon paprika, 1 tablespoon olive oil.

- Directions: In a small bowl, combine soy sauce, cocoa powder, cumin, chili powder, and paprika to make a marinade. Place the beef strips in the marinade and let them sit for 15-20 minutes. Heat olive oil in a skillet or wok over medium-high heat. Add the marinated beef and stir-fry for 3-4 minutes, until browned. Add broccoli, bell pepper, and carrots to the skillet and continue stir-frying for another 4-5 minutes, until the vegetables are tender-crisp and the beef is cooked through. Serve hot.

Miso-Glazed Salmon with Roasted Carrots:

- Ingredients: 4 salmon fillets (6 ounces each), 2 tablespoons white miso paste, 1 tablespoon honey, 1 tablespoon low-sodium soy sauce, 2 cloves garlic (minced), 1 tablespoon grated fresh ginger, 1 tablespoon sesame oil, 4 large carrots (peeled and cut into sticks), 1 tablespoon olive oil, salt, and pepper to taste.

- Directions: Preheat the oven to 400°F (200°C). In a small bowl, whisk together miso paste, honey, soy sauce, minced garlic, grated ginger, and sesame oil. Place the salmon fillets on a baking sheet and brush the miso glaze evenly over the top. Toss the carrot sticks with olive oil, salt, and pepper, then spread them around the salmon on the baking sheet. Roast for about 12-15 minutes, or until the salmon is cooked through and the carrots are tender. Serve hot.

Mediterranean Tuna Salad:

- Ingredients: 2 cans tuna (drained), 1 cup diced cucumber, 1 cup diced cherry tomatoes, 1/2 cup sliced Kalamata olives, 1/4 cup diced red onion, 2 tablespoons chopped fresh parsley, juice of 1 lemon, 2 tablespoons extra virgin olive oil, salt, and pepper to taste.

- Directions: In a large bowl, combine tuna, cucumber, cherry tomatoes, Kalamata olives, red onion, and parsley. In a small bowl, whisk together lemon juice, extra virgin olive oil, salt, and pepper to make a dressing. Pour the dressing over the tuna mixture and toss to coat. Serve chilled.

Pineapple Salsa with Baked Mackerel:

- Ingredients: 4 mackerel fillets (6 ounces each), 2 cups diced fresh pineapple, 1/2 cup diced red bell pepper, 1/4 cup diced red onion, 2 tablespoons chopped fresh cilantro, juice of 1 lime, salt, and pepper to taste.

- Directions: Preheat the oven to 375°F (190°C). Place the mackerel fillets on a baking sheet lined with parchment paper. Season with salt and pepper. Bake for about 12-15 minutes, or until the fish is cooked through. In a bowl, combine diced pineapple, red bell pepper, red onion, cilantro, lime juice, salt, and pepper to make the salsa. Serve the baked mackerel topped with the pineapple salsa.

Quinoa-Stuffed Tomatoes:

- Ingredients: 4 large tomatoes, 1 cup cooked quinoa, 1/2 cup crumbled feta cheese, 1/4 cup chopped fresh basil, 2 tablespoons extra virgin olive oil, salt, and pepper to taste.

- Directions: Preheat the oven to 400°F (200°C). Slice off the tops of the tomatoes and scoop out the seeds and pulp. In a bowl, combine cooked quinoa, feta cheese, chopped basil, olive oil, salt, and pepper. Stuff the tomato shells with the quinoa mixture. Place the stuffed tomatoes in a baking dish and bake for about 15-20 minutes, or until the tomatoes are tender. Serve warm.

Grilled Salmon with Spinach and Broccoli

Ingredients:

- 4 salmon fillets

- 2 cups of fresh spinach

- 2 cups of broccoli florets

- 1 tablespoon of extra-virgin olive oil

- Salt and pepper to taste

Directions:

1. Preheat the grill to medium-high heat.

2. Season the salmon fillets with salt and pepper.

3. Grill the salmon for about 4-5 minutes per side, until cooked through.

4. In a separate pan, heat the olive oil and sauté the spinach and broccoli until tender.

5. Serve the grilled salmon on a bed of sautéed spinach and broccoli. Enjoy!

Approximately 350 per serving

Tomato and Tuna Salad

Ingredients:

- 2 cans of tuna (in water)

- 2 cups of cherry tomatoes, halved

- 1 cup of diced carrots

- 1 tablespoon of lemon juice

- 2 tablespoons of extra-virgin olive oil

- Salt and pepper to taste

Directions:

1. In a bowl, combine the tuna, cherry tomatoes, and diced carrots.

2. Drizzle the lemon juice and olive oil over the mixture.

3. Season with salt and pepper, and toss to combine.

4. Serve the tomato and tuna salad chilled. It makes a refreshing and nutritious dinner option.

Calories: Approximately 200 per serving

Orange-Glazed Mackerel with Roasted Carrots

Ingredients:

- 4 mackerel fillets

- 4 medium carrots, peeled and sliced

- Juice and zest of 1 orange

- 2 tablespoons of honey

- 1 tablespoon of olive oil

- Salt and pepper to taste

Directions:

1. Preheat the oven to 400°F (200°C).

2. In a small bowl, mix the orange juice, orange zest, honey, olive oil, salt, and pepper to make the glaze.

3. Place the sliced carrots on a baking sheet and drizzle with half of the glaze.

4. Roast the carrots in the oven for about 20-25 minutes, until tender.

5. Meanwhile, season the mackerel fillets with salt and pepper, and brush them with the remaining glaze.

6. Grill or pan-fry the mackerel fillets for about 3-4 minutes per side, until cooked through.

7. Serve the orange-glazed mackerel with roasted carrots for a flavorful and satisfying dinner.

Calories: Approximately 400 per serving

Sardine and Spinach Stir-Fry

Ingredients:

- 2 cans of sardines (in olive oil), drained

- 4 cups of fresh spinach leaves

- 2 cloves of garlic, minced

- 1 tablespoon of soy sauce

- 1 tablespoon of sesame oil

- Red pepper flakes (optional)

- Cooked brown rice (optional, for serving)

Directions:

1. Heat the sesame oil in a pan over medium heat.

2. Add the minced garlic and sauté for about 1 minute until fragrant.

3. Add the sardines and spinach to the pan, and stir-fry until the spinach wilts.

4. Stir in the soy sauce and red pepper flakes (if desired), and cook for an additional minute.

5. Serve the sardine and spinach stir-fry over cooked brown rice or enjoy it on its own.

Calories: Approximately 250 per serving

Scan the photo here

Roasted Salmon with Citrus Glaze:

- Ingredients:

  - 4 salmon fillets (6 ounces each)

  - 1/4 cup freshly squeezed orange juice

  - 1/4 cup freshly squeezed lemon juice

  - 2 tablespoons honey

  - 2 cloves garlic, minced

- Salt and pepper to taste

- Directions:

  1. Preheat the oven to 400°F (200°C).

  2. In a small bowl, whisk together the orange juice, lemon juice, honey, minced garlic, salt, and pepper.

  3. Place the salmon fillets on a baking sheet lined with parchment paper.

  4. Brush the citrus glaze over the salmon fillets.

  5. Bake for 12-15 minutes, or until the salmon is cooked through and flakes easily with a fork.

- Description: This flavorful salmon dish is glazed with a tangy citrus sauce, giving it a refreshing and zesty taste. The high omega-3 fatty acids in salmon provide anti-inflammatory benefits.

- Cooking time: 12-15 minutes

- Calories: Approximately 300 per serving

- Tip: For quicker preparation, you can marinate the salmon in the citrus glaze for 30 minutes before baking to enhance the flavors.

Quinoa and Vegetable Stir-Fry:

- Ingredients:

  - 2 cups cooked quinoa

  - 1 cup broccoli florets

  - 1 cup sliced bell peppers

  - 1 cup sliced carrots

  - 1 cup snap peas

  - 2 cloves garlic, minced

  - 2 tablespoons low-sodium soy sauce

  - 1 tablespoon olive oil

  - Salt and pepper to taste

- Directions:

1. Heat olive oil in a large skillet or wok over medium-high heat.

2. Add the minced garlic and sauté for 1 minute until fragrant.

3. Add the broccoli florets, bell peppers, carrots, and snap peas to the skillet and stir-fry for 4-5 minutes, or until the vegetables are crisp-tender.

4. Stir in the cooked quinoa and soy sauce, and season with salt and pepper.

5. Continue to stir-fry for another 2-3 minutes until everything is well combined.

- Description: This vibrant stir-fry combines nutrient-rich quinoa with a colorful mix of vegetables, creating a delicious and satisfying meal. Quinoa is a great source of plant-based protein and contains anti-inflammatory properties.

- Cooking time: 10-12 minutes

- Calories: Approximately 250 per serving

- Tip: To save time, you can use pre-cooked quinoa or leftover quinoa from a previous meal.

Baked Mackerel with Tomato Salsa:

- Ingredients:

  - 4 mackerel fillets (6 ounces each)

  - 2 cups diced tomatoes

  - 1/2 cup diced red onion

  - 1/4 cup chopped fresh parsley

  - 2 tablespoons extra virgin olive oil

  - 2 tablespoons lemon juice

  - Salt and pepper to taste

- Directions:

  1. Preheat the oven to 375°F (190°C).

  2. Place the mackerel fillets on a baking sheet lined with parchment paper.

  3. Season the fillets with salt, pepper, and a drizzle of olive oil.

  4. In a bowl, combine the diced tomatoes, red onion, parsley, olive oil, lemon juice, salt, and pepper to make the tomato salsa.

5. Spoon the salsa over the mackerel fillets.

6. Bake for 15-18 minutes, or until the mackerel is cooked through and flakes easily.

- Description: This baked mackerel dish is paired with a refreshing tomato salsa, adding bright flavors to the tender fish. Mackerel is rich in omega-3 fatty acids, making it an excellent choice for an anti-inflammatory diet.

- Cooking time: 15-18 minutes

- Calories: Approximately 200 per serving

- Tip: Prepare the tomato salsa in advance and refrigerate it to save time when assembling the dish.

Cocoa-Spiced Beef Stir-Fry with Vegetables:

Scan the photo here

- Ingredients:

  - 1pound beef sirloin, thinly sliced

  - 2 cups broccoli florets

  - 1 cup sliced bell peppers

  - 1 cup sliced carrots

  - 2 tablespoons low-sodium soy sauce

  - 1 tablespoon unsweetened cocoa powder

  - 1 teaspoon ground cumin

  - 1/2 teaspoon chili powder

  - 1/2 teaspoon paprika

  - 1 tablespoon olive oil

  - Salt and pepper to taste

- Directions:

  1. In a small bowl, combine the soy sauce, cocoa powder, cumin, chili powder, paprika, salt, and pepper to make a marinade.

  2. Place the beef slices in the marinade and let them sit for 15-20 minutes.

  3. Heat olive oil in a skillet or wok over medium-high heat.

  4. Add the marinated beef slices and stir-fry for 3-4 minutes, or until browned.

5. Add the broccoli florets, bell peppers, and carrots to the skillet and continue stir-frying for another 4-5 minutes until the vegetables are tender-crisp and the beef is cooked to your desired doneness.

- Description: This cocoa-spiced beef stir-fry combines tender beef with a blend of spices and colorful vegetables, resulting in a savory and satisfying meal. Cocoa powder adds a unique depth of flavor and antioxidants to the dish.

- Cooking time: 10-12 minutes

- Calories: Approximately 300 per serving

- Tip: To save time on slicing the beef, you can purchase pre-sliced beef sirloin from the grocery store.

Grilled Tuna Steak with Pineapple Salsa:

- Ingredients:

  - 4 tuna steaks (6 ounces each)

  - 2 cups diced fresh pineapple

  - 1/2 cup diced red bell pepper

  - 1/4 cup diced red onion

  - 2 tablespoons chopped fresh cilantro

  - Juice of 1 lime

  - Salt and pepper to taste

- Directions:

  1. Preheat the grill to medium-high heat.

  2. Season the tuna steaks with salt and pepper.

  3. Grill the tuna steaks for 3-4 minutes per side, or until cooked to your desired level of doneness.

  4. In a bowl, combine the diced pineapple, red bell pepper, red onion, cilantro, lime juice, salt, and pepper to make the pineapple salsa.

  5. Serve the grilled tuna steaks topped with the pineapple salsa.

- Description: This grilled

tuna steak is complemented by a tangy and refreshing pineapple salsa, creating a delightful combination of flavors. The tuna steak is rich in omega-3 fatty acids, while the pineapple adds a touch of sweetness and vitamin C to the dish.

- Cooking time: 8-10 minutes

- Calories: Approximately 250 per serving

- Tip: To speed up the grilling process, make sure the grill is preheated and properly oiled before placing the tuna steaks on it.

These dinner recipes offer a range of flavors and nutritious ingredients to support an anti-inflammatory diet. Enjoy the benefits of these delicious meals while taking care of your health in a fun and relaxing way.

28 Days-Meal Plan

Day 1:

- Breakfast: Fresh Berry Parfait

- Lunch: Avocado Toast

- Dinner: Baked Salmon with Roasted Vegetables

- Snack: Cucumber Hummus Bites

Day 2:

- Breakfast: Chia Pudding

- Lunch: Greek Yogurt Dip with Veggies

- Dinner: Spinach and Quinoa Stuffed Bell Peppers

- Snack: Apple Slices with Almond Butter

Day 3:

- Breakfast: Pineapple and Blueberry Smoothie

- Lunch: Rice Cake with Smashed Avocado

- Dinner: Tomato Basil Chicken Skewers

- Snack: Fresh Berry Parfait

Day 4:

- Breakfast: Fresh Berry Parfait

- Lunch: Mediterranean Tuna Salad

- Dinner: Cocoa-Spiced Beef Stir-Fry

- Snack: Trail Mix

Day 5:

- Breakfast: Avocado Toast

- Lunch: Cucumber Hummus Bites

- Dinner: Baked Mackerel with Tomato Salsa

- Snack: Greek Yogurt Dip with Veggies

Day 6:

- Breakfast: Chia Pudding

- Lunch: Greek Yogurt Berry Popsicles

- Dinner: Quinoa-Stuffed Tomatoes

- Snack: Apple Slices with Almond Butter

Day 7:

- Breakfast: Pineapple and Blueberry Smoothie

- Lunch: Fresh Berry Parfait

- Dinner: Grilled Tuna Steak with Pineapple Salsa

- Snack: Rice Cake with Smashed Avocado

Day 8:

- Breakfast: Avocado Toast

- Lunch: Tomato and Tuna Salad

- Dinner: Grilled Salmon with Spinach and Broccoli

- Snack: Cucumber Hummus Bites

Day 9:

- Breakfast: Chia Pudding

- Lunch: Greek Yogurt Dip with Veggies

- Dinner: Miso-Glazed Salmon with Roasted Carrots

- Snack: Apple Slices with Almond Butter

Day 10:

- Breakfast: Pineapple and Blueberry Smoothie

- Lunch: Rice Cake with Smashed Avocado

- Dinner: Sardine and Spinach Stir-Fry

- Snack: Greek Yogurt Berry Popsicles

Day 11:

- Breakfast: Fresh Berry Parfait

- Lunch: Mediterranean Tuna Salad

- Dinner: Quinoa and Vegetable Stir-Fry

- Snack: Trail Mix

Day 12:

- Breakfast: Avocado Toast

- Lunch: Cucumber Hummus Bites

- Dinner: Baked Salmon with Roasted Vegetables

- Snack: Apple Slices with Almond Butter

Day 13:

- Breakfast: Chia Pudding

- Lunch: Greek Yogurt Dip with Veggies

- Dinner: Cocoa-Spiced Beef Stir-Fry

- Snack: Fresh Berry Parfait

Day 14:

- Breakfast: Pineapple and Blueberry Smoothie

- Lunch: Fresh Berry Parfait

- Dinner: Grilled Tuna Steak with Pineapple Salsa

- Snack: Rice Cake with Smashed Avocado

- Snack: Trail Mix

Day 15:

- Breakfast: Avocado Toast

- Lunch: Tomato and Tuna Salad

- Dinner: Grilled Salmon with Spinach and Broccoli

- Snack: Cucumber Hummus Bites

Day 16:

- Breakfast: Chia Pudding

- Lunch: Greek Yogurt Dip with Veggies

- Dinner: Miso-Glazed Salmon with Roasted Carrots

- Snack: Apple Slices with Almond Butter

Day 17:

- Breakfast: Pineapple and Blueberry Smoothie

- Lunch: Rice Cake with Smashed Avocado

- Dinner: Sardine and Spinach Stir-Fry

- Snack: Greek Yogurt Berry Popsicles

Day 18:

- Breakfast: Fresh Berry Parfait

- Lunch: Mediterranean Tuna Salad

- Dinner: Quinoa and Vegetable Stir-Fry

Day 19:

- Breakfast: Avocado Toast

- Lunch: Cucumber Hummus Bites

- Dinner: Baked Salmon with Roasted Vegetables

- Snack: Apple Slices with Almond Butter

Day 20:

- Breakfast: Chia Pudding

- Lunch: Greek Yogurt Dip with Veggies

- Dinner: Cocoa-Spiced Beef Stir-Fry

- Snack: Fresh Berry Parfait

Day 21:

- Breakfast: Pineapple and Blueberry Smoothie

- Lunch: Fresh Berry Parfait

- Dinner: Grilled Tuna Steak with Pineapple Salsa

- Snack: Rice Cake with Smashed Avocado

Day 22:

- Breakfast: Avocado Toast

- Lunch: Tomato and Tuna Salad

- Dinner: Grilled Salmon with Spinach and Broccoli

- Snack: Cucumber Hummus Bites

Day 23:

- Breakfast: Chia Pudding

- Lunch: Greek Yogurt Dip with Veggies

- Dinner: Miso-Glazed Salmon with Roasted Carrots

- Snack: Apple Slices with Almond Butter

Day 24:

- Breakfast: Pineapple and Blueberry Smoothie

- Lunch: Rice Cake with Smashed Avocado

- Dinner: Sardine and Spinach Stir-Fry

- Snack: Greek Yogurt Berry Popsicles

Day 25:

- Breakfast: Fresh Berry Parfait

- Lunch: Mediterranean Tuna Salad

- Dinner: Quinoa and Vegetable Stir-Fry

- Snack: Trail Mix

Day 26:

- Breakfast: Avocado Toast

- Lunch: Cucumber Hummus Bites

- Dinner: Baked Salmon with Roasted Vegetables

- Snack: Apple Slices with Almond Butter

Day 27:

- Breakfast: Chia Pudding

- Lunch: Greek Yogurt Dip with Veggies

- Dinner: Cocoa-Spiced Beef Stir-Fry

- Snack: Fresh Berry Parfait

Day 28:

- Breakfast: Pineapple and Blueberry Smoothie

- Lunch: Fresh Berry Parfait

- Dinner: Grilled Tuna Steak with Pineapple Salsa

- Snack: Rice Cake with Smashed Avocado

Remember to listen to your body and make any necessary modifications to accommodate your dietary needs and

preferences. Enjoy your meals and have a healthy and delicious 28-day journey!

BONUS 2

Thank you for purchasing our Anti-inflammatory Diet Cookbook. Inside, you'll find four **QR** codes, each containing **100** video recipes, totaling **400** easy and quick recipes. Each video includes step-by-step instructions for preparing delicious meals.

Enjoy your culinary journey and embrace a healthier lifestyle!

400 Video-Recipe

Conclusion

Dear Reader,

As we conclude this journey through the pages of the "Anti-Inflammatory Diet Cookbook for Beginners," I want to extend my heartfelt gratitude for joining me on this transformative path towards better health and wellness. Your commitment to exploring the power of an anti-inflammatory diet is commendable, and I hope this cookbook has served as a valuable resource on your journey.

The benefits of embracing an anti-inflammatory diet are multifaceted and impactful. By incorporating nourishing, whole foods abundant in antioxidants, essential nutrients, and anti-inflammatory properties, you're not just shaping your diet – you're enhancing your overall well-being. Through this approach, many experience reduced inflammation, improved digestion, enhanced energy levels, and even better mental clarity. Moreover, this dietary shift often contributes to weight management and supports a stronger immune system.

This cookbook is crafted with beginners in mind, but the principles of an anti-inflammatory diet are suitable for anyone seeking a healthier lifestyle. Whether you're managing specific health conditions, looking to prevent diseases, or simply aiming for increased vitality, this diet can be a pivotal step in achieving your wellness goals.

Remember, perseverance is key. Embracing a new dietary regimen can sometimes pose challenges, but your dedication to making positive changes in your life is commendable. Stay committed to your goals, even on days when it feels challenging, as the long-term benefits of an anti-inflammatory diet are worth the effort.

As you continue your journey towards better health, I encourage you to stay curious, explore new recipes, and remain open to the transformative power of food. Your dedication to nurturing your body and mind through wholesome, anti-inflammatory meals is a testament to your commitment to living your best life.

Once again, I express my sincere thanks for choosing this cookbook as your guide. May your path be filled with delicious, nourishing meals that fuel your body and inspire your spirit.

With heartfelt gratitude,